STRONGER FOOD AND DRUG REGULATORY SYSTEMS ABROAD

Committee on Stronger Food and Drug Regulatory Systems Abroad

Board on Global Health

Health and Medicine Division

Gillian J. Buckley and Catherine E. Woteki, *Editors*

A Consensus Study Report of
The National Academies of
SCIENCES · ENGINEERING · MEDICINE

THE NATIONAL ACADEMIES PRESS
Washington, DC
www.nap.edu

THE NATIONAL ACADEMIES PRESS 500 Fifth Street, NW Washington, DC 20001

This activity was supported by contracts between the National Academy of Sciences and the Food and Drug Administration (#10004259). Any opinions, findings, conclusions, or recommendations expressed in this publication do not necessarily reflect the views of any organization or agency that provided support for the project.

International Standard Book Number-13: 978-0-309-67043-2
International Standard Book Number-10: 0-309-67043-8
Digital Object Identifier: https://doi.org/10.17226/25651

Additional copies of this publication are available from the National Academies Press, 500 Fifth Street, NW, Keck 360, Washington, DC 20001; (800) 624-6242 or (202) 334-3313; http://www.nap.edu.

Printed in the United States of America

Suggested citation: National Academies of Sciences, Engineering, and Medicine. 2020. *Stronger food and drug regulatory systems abroad.* Washington, DC: The National Academies Press. https://doi.org/10.17226/25651.

The National Academies of
SCIENCES · ENGINEERING · MEDICINE

The **National Academy of Sciences** was established in 1863 by an Act of Congress, signed by President Lincoln, as a private, nongovernmental institution to advise the nation on issues related to science and technology. Members are elected by their peers for outstanding contributions to research. Dr. Marcia McNutt is president.

The **National Academy of Engineering** was established in 1964 under the charter of the National Academy of Sciences to bring the practices of engineering to advising the nation. Members are elected by their peers for extraordinary contributions to engineering. Dr. John L. Anderson is president.

The **National Academy of Medicine** (formerly the Institute of Medicine) was established in 1970 under the charter of the National Academy of Sciences to advise the nation on medical and health issues. Members are elected by their peers for distinguished contributions to medicine and health. Dr. Victor J. Dzau is president.

The three Academies work together as the **National Academies of Sciences, Engineering, and Medicine** to provide independent, objective analysis and advice to the nation and conduct other activities to solve complex problems and inform public policy decisions. The National Academies also encourage education and research, recognize outstanding contributions to knowledge, and increase public understanding in matters of science, engineering, and medicine.

Learn more about the National Academies of Sciences, Engineering, and Medicine at **www.nationalacademies.org**.

COMMITTEE ON STRONGER FOOD AND DRUG REGULATORY SYSTEMS ABROAD

CATHERINE E. WOTEKI (*Chair*), Professor, Iowa State University
LYSTRA ANTOINE, CEO of Global Food Safety Partnership, World Bank
MIKEL ARRIOLA, former Federal Commissioner, COFEPRIS; former General Director, Mexican Institute of Social Security
MARIA ELENA BOTTAZZI, Associate Dean and Professor, National School of Tropical Medicine, Baylor College of Medicine
JULIE CASWELL, Distinguished Professor Emeritus, University of Massachusetts Amherst
CLARE NARROD, Director of Risk Analysis Program, Joint Institute for Food Safety and Applied Nutrition, University of Maryland
JONATHAN QUICK, Senior Fellow Emeritus, Management Sciences for Health
JOSHUA SHARFSTEIN, Vice Dean and Professor, Johns Hopkins Bloomberg School of Public Health
MARKUS TAUSSIG, Associate Professor, Rutgers Business School
RAYMOND WIGENGE, former Director of Food and Safety, Tanzania Food and Drug Authority
VERONIKA WIRTZ, Associate Professor, Department of Global Health, Boston University School of Public Health
PRASHANT YADAV, Visiting Fellow, Center for Global Development; Affiliate Professor of Technology & Operations Management, INSEAD

Health and Medicine Division Staff

GILLIAN J. BUCKLEY, Study Director
ROMY NATHAN, Program Officer (*from August 2019*)
AMBAR SAEED, Research Associate
SARAH ANNE NEW, Senior Program Assistant (*until April 2019*)
MARGARET McFARLAND, Senior Program Assistant (*from May 2019*)
JULIE PAVLIN, Director, Board on Global Health

National Academy of Medicine Fellow in Pharmacy

DIMA QATO, Associate Professor, University of Illinois at Chicago College of Pharmacy

Reviewers

This Consensus Study Report was reviewed in draft form by individuals chosen for their diverse perspectives and technical expertise. The purpose of this independent review is to provide candid and critical comments that will assist the National Academies of Sciences, Engineering, and Medicine in making each published report as sound as possible and to ensure that it meets the institutional standards for quality, objectivity, evidence, and responsiveness to the study charge. The review comments and draft manuscript remain confidential to protect the integrity of the deliberative process.

We thank the following individuals for their review of this report:

JIE BAI, Harvard Kennedy School
ANA MARISA CORDERO, Inter-American Institute for Cooperation on Agriculture
KELLEY CORMIER, U.S. Agency for International Development
KENNETH HARTIGAN-GO, Asian Institute of Management Philippines
STEVEN M. JAFFEE, University of Maryland
PATRICK LUKULAY, Technology Solutions for Global Health
JOHN T. MONAHAN, Georgetown University
JUDE NWOKIKE, United States Pharmacopeial Convention
ALAIN PRAT, The Global Fund to Fight AIDS, Tuberculosis and Malaria

CARLOS SANTOS-BURGOA, The George Washington University
ANDY STERGACHIS, University of Washington
JOSE VICENTE COTO UGARTE, Pan American Health Organization

Although the reviewers listed above provided many constructive comments and suggestions, they were not asked to endorse the conclusions or recommendations of this report nor did they see the final draft before its release. The review of this report was overseen by **JIM E. RIVIERE,** North Carolina State University and Kansas State University, and **LYNN R. GOLDMAN,** The George Washington University. They were responsible for making certain that an independent examination of this report was carried out in accordance with the standards of the National Academies and that all review comments were carefully considered. Responsibility for the final content rests entirely with the authoring committee and the National Academies.

Acknowledgments

This consensus study report is a product of the cooperation and contributions of many people. The committee and staff are especially grateful for the support of the National Academies of Sciences, Engineering, and Medicine staff, especially Daniel Bearss, Clyde Behney, Jeanay Butler, Anna Isabel Camilo Javier, Daniel Cesnalis, Kierra Chinn, Julie Eubank, Greta Gorman, Nicole Joy, Stephanie Miceli, Rebecca Morgan, Tina Seliber, Lauren Shern, Elizabeth Tyson, Julie Wiltshire, and Taryn Young. We also specially thank Rebekah Hutton for designing the report cover.

The committee's overseas workshop went smoothly thanks to the warm hospitality from the National Academy of Sciences of Costa Rica, especially Walter Fernandez, Pedro Leon, and Dayana Mora.

Many people kindly introduced the Health and Medicine Division staff to key speakers. They are particularly grateful to Javier Guzman, Analia Porrás, and Mike Ward.

The committee thanks all the speakers and moderators who participated in committee meetings, as well as others who provided information, input, and assistance. They include Pawan Agarwal, Jean Carlo Apuy, Dirceu Barbano, Jarbas Barbosa, Rommel Anibal Betancourt Herrera, Marisa Caipo, Renata Clarke, Monique Collaço de Moraes Stávale, Ana Marisa Cordero, Kelley Cormier, Santiago Cornejo, Jose Vicente Coto Ugarte, Lissy Cruz, Tatiana Cruz Ramirez, Rivelino Flores, Juan Carlos Galarza, Iris Galeano, Delia Grace, Nuri Gras, Kenneth Hartigan-Go, Lisa Indar, Steven Jaffee, Barbara Kowalcyk, Larry Liberti, Lisa Ludeman, Mac Lumpkin, Gugu Mahlangu, Emilio Medina, Mario Montero, Uy Hong

Nguyen, Jude Nwokike, Carolina Paz, Mayra Perez-Tapia, Anban Pillay, Elizabeth Pisani, Lembit Rago, Maria Angelica Sanchez-Herrera, Carlos Santos Burgoa, Katherine Serrano, Dilip Shah, Paula Vargas, Dali Young, and Ana Gabriel Zuniga.

We thank Hudu Mogtari of the African Union's New Partnership for Africa's Development program for his willingness to serve on the committee. Mr. Mogtari was obliged to resign from the committee before participating in any deliberations because of other commitments.

Finally, particular thanks to the U.S. Food and Drug Administration for generously funding this project.

Contents

APPENDIXES

Boxes, Figures, and Tables

BOXES

FIGURES

TABLES

Acronyms and Abbreviations

ADDO	Accredited Drug Dispensing Outlet
AIDS	acquired immunodeficiency syndrome
APEC	Asia-Pacific Economic Cooperation
ASEAN	Association of Southeast Asian Nations
AUDA	African Union Development Agency
CDC	U.S. Centers for Disease Control and Prevention
EFSA	European Food Safety Authority
EMA	European Medicines Agency
FAO	Food and Agriculture Organization of the United Nations
FDA	U.S. Food and Drug Administration
FSIS	Food Safety and Inspection Service
GAP	Good Agricultural Practices
GBT	Global Benchmarking Tool
GFSI	Global Food Safety Initiative
GFSP	Global Food Safety Partnership
HACCP	Hazard Analysis and Critical Control Point
HHS	U.S. Department of Health and Human Services
HIV	human immunodeficiency virus

ICDRA	International Conference of Drug Regulatory Authorities
ICH	International Council for Harmonization of Technical Requirements for Pharmaceuticals for Human Use
ICMRA	International Coalition of Medicines Regulatory Authorities
IFC	International Finance Corporation
IFPTI	International Food Protection Training Institute
ILSI	International Life Sciences Institute
IMDRF	International Medical Device Regulators Forum
IMF	International Monetary Fund
INFOSAN	International Food Safety Authorities Network
IOM	Institute of Medicine
ISO	International Organization for Standardization
JIFSAN	Joint Institute for Food Safety and Applied Nutrition
NAFDAC	National Agency for Food and Drug Administration and Control
NCD	noncommunicable disease
NEPAD	New Partnership for Africa's Development
NIH	National Institutes of Health
OECD	Organisation for Economic Co-operation and Development
OIE	World Organisation for Animal Health
PEPFAR	The President's Emergency Plan for AIDS Relief
PVS	Performance of Veterinary Services
SADCAS	Southern Africa Development Community Accreditation Service
UN	United Nations
UNIDO	United Nations Industrial Development Organization
USAID	U.S. Agency for International Development
USDA	U.S. Department of Agriculture
WHA	World Health Assembly
WHO	World Health Organization
WTO	World Trade Organization

Summary[1]

Ensuring the safety of food and the quality and safety of medicines in a country is an important role of government, described by the World Health Organization (WHO) as an essential public health function. It is a technical and labor-intensive job, made more complicated by global manufacturing and international trade. Occasionally, product safety scares in the United States draw attention to the role of the U.S. Food and Drug and Administration (FDA), but for the most part, the regulation of food and medicines is taken for granted because it works well. The same cannot be said in most low- and middle-income countries. By recent estimates, unsafe food kills over 400,000 people a year, a third of them children under 5, mostly in low- and middle-income countries; every year poor quality medicines cause about 70,000 excess deaths from childhood pneumonia and roughly 8,500 to 20,000 malaria deaths in sub-Saharan Africa alone.

These and similar problems are of special concern to the FDA Office of Global Policy and Strategy[2] as it is charged with improving capacity of the agency's foreign counterpart offices and increasing understanding of the importance of regulatory systems for public health, development, and trade. This mission influenced the agency's commission of the 2012 Institute of Medicine report on regulatory systems, *Ensuring Safe Food and Medical Products Through Stronger Regulatory Systems Abroad.* Among other things, the report outlines strategies to secure international supply chains,

[1] References are not included in the report summary. Please view the body of the report for a full list of works cited.

[2] Formerly called the Office of International Programs.

emphasizes capacity building and support for surveillance in low- and middle-income countries, and explores ways to facilitate work sharing among food and medical product regulatory agencies (hereafter, regulatory agencies).

Circumstances for regulators have evolved since 2012, as has the broader context of global health and development. With this in mind, the FDA Office of Global Policy and Strategy commissioned this study to clarify how such transitions affect the way regulators work, to promote understanding of the importance of regulatory systems, and to increase scientific robustness at regulatory agencies.

The committee recognizes the responsibility regulators have for the products in their market, while also emphasizing that these agencies do not operate in a vacuum. Therefore, the report gives considerable emphasis to actions at the global and national levels that foster the ability of a regulatory agency to function well. The report starts with analysis of global programs and trends, moving to increasingly narrow sub-divisions. As Table S-1 shows, recommendations start at the global level, then move to changes at the level of the national government. The last group of recommendations are made at the level of the regulatory agency, suggesting an agenda for regulatory agencies and cooperation among countries.

This report sets out a strategy to support good-quality, wholesome food and safe, effective medical products around the world. Its goal is to build on the momentum for strengthening regulatory systems and to set a course for sustainability and continued progress.

REGULATORY SYSTEMS, GLOBAL HEALTH, AND DEVELOPMENT

Health in low- and middle-income countries has improved over the last two decades. Child mortality and infectious disease prevalence have fallen; nutrition has improved. While bilateral, multilateral, and private donors deserve credit for this progress, it is also a function of increasing global prosperity and national investments in health systems and other social programs. By 2020, about half the world will live in a middle-class household. This change has implications for governments, as members of the middle class are better able to demand safe food and health services. But public services in most of the world are not keeping pace with that change. Safe food and good-quality medicines are a precondition to successful development, since a growing demand for these products is a consequence of progress.

Strengthening regulatory systems is important for continued global prosperity and progress in health. It also requires a common understanding of the regulatory process. Risk-based decision making, including the continuous and iterative assessment of risk, is the cornerstone of this process.

TABLE S-1
Overview of Report Organization and Recommendations by Topic and Intended Actors

Level of Action	Topic	Actors	Recommendation
Global	Food safety	FAO and WHO	Recommendation 2-1: The Food and Agriculture Organization of the United Nations (FAO) and the World Health Organization (WHO) should convene biennial meetings for food safety regulators similar to the International Conference of Drug Regulatory Authorities.
	Medical products	WHO	Recommendation 3-2: The World Health Organization should expand prequalification to include treatments for cancer, diabetes, and other diseases with a high global burden.
	Global health and develop-ment	Donor organiza-tions work-ing in health and develop-ment	Recommendation 3-1: Development partners, including multilateral and bilateral donors and private philanthropic organizations, should encourage countries' participation in regulatory benchmarking assessments, the development of institutional development plans, and reports on progress against those plans. To this end, assistance should be targeted to priorities identified in benchmarking assessments and the related institutional development plans.
			Recommendation 3-3: Development partners, including multilateral and bilateral donors and private philanthropic organizations, should support countries and regional organization in pursuing greater collaboration for regulating food and medical products. This collaboration can include harmonization and mutual recognition of data or standards, equivalence agreements, and regulatory reliance.
			Recommendation 3-4: Development finance institutions such as the United States International Development Finance Corporation, the International Finance Corporation (IFC), the UK CDC Group, and the European development finance banks should create vehicles to finance producers, distributors, and retailers in low- and middle-income countries interested in meeting regulatory standards. This would involve advisory services and, when appropriate, concessional financing.
			Recommendation 3-5: The United States International Development Finance Corporation, the International Finance Corporation (IFC), the UK CDC Group, and the European development finance banks should provide advisory services and concessional financing to manufacturers of quality and safety screening technologies to optimize manufacturing and create stronger distribution systems in low- and middle-income countries.
		NIH, FDA, and USAID	Recommendation 3-6: The National Institutes of Health, in collaboration with the U.S. Food and Drug Administration and the U.S. Agency for International Development, should develop a network of Global Centers of Excellence in Regulatory Science for research and capacity building to address the challenges of food and drug safety in low- and middle-income countries.

continued

TABLE S-1 Continued

Level of Action	Topic	Actors	Recommendation
National	Government and financing	National governments, their leaders	Recommendation 4-1: National governments should guarantee in legislation that national regulatory agencies be independent and financially viable, with statutes that encourage cooperation with other agencies and require a scientific basis for decision making.
Agency	Risk-based regulation, communication, and information	Food and drug regulatory agencies	Recommendation 5-1: National regulatory authorities should take a risk-based approach to the regulation of food and medicines. This includes: a. Developing effective data systems to systematically identify areas of greatest risk; b. Participating in research, data sharing, technology adoption, and training activities with international partners; c. Growing capacity to assess the health and economic impacts of regulation, and using this information to inform actions to protect public health; d. Communicating about risks, including the uncertainty around them, especially during crisis; and e. Communicating the ways regulation improves quality, safety, and access, using different strategies to convey this information to government leaders, regulated industry, and the public.
	Informal markets		Recommendation 5-2: National regulatory agencies should use evidence to guide strategies to reduce the risk posed by informal markets. Strategies to consider include accreditation or licensing to formalize sellers, consumer education, and increasing competition from regulated products.
	Management and collaboration		Recommendation 5-3: National regulatory authorities should take advantage of global tools to support regulatory actions. Resources from United Nations agencies, including World Health Organization prequalification and Codex standards, are examples of such tools, as are the third-party standards increasingly used in food and agriculture.
			Recommendation 5-4: National regulatory authorities should determine which functions are most effectively and efficiently carried out directly by the agency and which can be delegated to state or local authorities; collaboration and data sharing among domestic agencies should be part of any delegation plan.

Data from and public consultation with a range of stakeholders, both domestically and internationally, are also crucial. International agreement on technical guidelines, requirements for registration, and the approach to inspections can control the regulatory burden on industry; it also reduces repetitive work. International collaboration has therefore been cited as a minimum function of the regulatory agency. There are many international venues for such collaboration; some are initiated by industry, others are the product of trade or bilateral relationships. A recent 2-year mapping exercise by the International Coalition of Medicines Regulatory Authorities led to comments on the overlapping objectives and confusing array of similar initiatives.

There is no comparable, international mapping of food safety programs, partly because there is no analogous international coalition of food regulators. This is unfortunate, as the modern food safety landscape is so complex that even people with the best knowledge of the system see only parts of it. It is also symptomatic of a larger problem, the absence of a standing international venue for food regulators to interact with their counterparts around the world. Such a convention is an investment in the efficiency of the various regional cooperatives and technical groups working in the field. Convening food regulators also supports emergency response, building relationships that regulators can draw on during a crisis.

Recommendation 2-1: The Food and Agriculture Organization of the United Nations (FAO) and the World Health Organization (WHO) should convene biennial meetings for food safety regulators similar to the International Conference of Drug Regulatory Authorities.

The increasing complexity of regulatory work and the interconnected nature of the food supply chain make it necessary for food regulators to have a standing, formal venue for exchange and cooperation. As the United Nations (UN) agencies responsible for global health and food security, the FAO and the WHO are the best choices to convene the meeting suggested.

GLOBAL EFFORTS TO STRENGTHEN REGULATORY SYSTEMS

Recent reports on falsified and substandard medicines and foodborne disease in low- and middle-income countries have drawn attention to the consequences of regulatory failures. Yet, much of the immediate reaction to such news has emphasized local solutions, from the need for consumers to demand food safety from their governments to the responsibility of governments to enforce regulations. While no one could deny the importance of the consumer, regulator, or political leader in solving these problems, their actions are of limited value if the global environment does not foster product safety. Part of this report discusses how circumstances beyond the policy of any country influence food and medical product systems.

The Role of Aid

Global health and development organizations have considerable power to influence policy in ways that encourage functional regulatory systems. Development aid is one important tool to this end. Since the 1990s, there has been concern that the manner in which aid is given can do unintentional harm to recipient countries. In an effort to avoid this harm, the Organisation for Economic Co-operation and Development (OECD) has set out principles of aid effectiveness, two of which are especially relevant to the discussion of building regulatory systems. One is the untying of aid, meaning the removal of conditions that require recipient countries to procure goods and services through the donor country. The other is institution building, meaning spending in ways that support organizations and capacity in the recipient country. Attention to regulatory systems advances both goals, building the institutions that protect product safety, thereby increasing options for local procurement.

A valid benchmarking tool can put clear parameters on the concept of building regulatory institutions, thereby making it more concrete, measurable, and attractive to donor investment. The WHO Global Benchmarking Tool is an assessment for agencies that regulate medical products. Benchmarking assessment involves independent evaluation on nine functions; results inform a 5-year institutional development plan, which in turn informs a strategy to improve on identified weaknesses. Benchmarking food systems is more complicated. Food safety involves a variety of different fields, and there are various benchmarking tools for plant and animal health, as well as a more comprehensive food system assessment from the WHO and the FAO.

The institutional development plans developed out of benchmarking assessments help translate the sometimes vague job of institution building into concrete measurable steps. This is not a benefit that can be realized if countries do not participate in the benchmarking assessment, however, making an incentive to participate especially valuable. Global health and development organizations, including UN agencies, development banks, bilateral donors, and private philanthropy (described increasingly as "development partners") all have a role to play in providing such incentive.

Recommendation 3-1: Development partners, including multilateral and bilateral donors and private philanthropic organizations, should encourage countries' participation in regulatory benchmarking

assessments, the development of institutional development plans, and reports on progress against those plans. To this end, assistance should be targeted to priorities identified in benchmarking assessments and the related institutional development plans.

The move toward universal health coverage means that countries are now responsible for the purchase of more and varied types of medicines. This puts a strain on health budgets, even more so in those middle-income countries transitioning away from donor procurement. An increased demand for medical products draws attention to the essential procurement question of value for money, something that can be difficult to judge, especially when products are imported.

The WHO Prequalification Program provides regulatory assessment, inspection, and ongoing quality control for certain medical products procured through UN agencies or other large donors. Though the WHO does not act as a supra-national regulator, prequalification can act as a proxy regulatory approval that helps manage the combination of limited regulatory capacity and foreign procurement. It also has an important capacity building element for both manufacturers and regulators. Regulators from advanced agencies and from agencies in the countries where prequalified products will be used work together on prequalification teams; the program has also shown positive spillover effects on manufacturing.

Recommendation 3-2: The World Health Organization should expand prequalification to include treatments for cancer, diabetes, and other diseases with a high global burden.

In its recent 5-year plan to build regulatory capacity, the WHO cited prequalification as a strategic priority. The committee commends this plan and encourages the WHO to look beyond those products associated with HIV, tuberculosis, and malaria in its expansion. The choice of products and the order in which they are added to the prequalification list are topics for further discussion. There is clear demand for any product where a third or more of the total market by volume is subject to global procurement. Review of the Global Burden of Disease data will also be important to this discussion, as will considerations for products with small but important markets. Biologic medicines present a particular challenge to regulators because of the complexity of manufacturing. Biologic treatments would also be good candidates as would anti-infectives since the risk of drug resistance makes the quality of these products a global public good.

Expansion of prequalification puts a financial burden on the WHO, and an increased demand for expertise from advanced regulatory agencies. The products included in prequalification to date are those procured by international agencies. Treatments for noncommunicable diseases are subject to national procurement, which cannot command the same negotiating power. Nevertheless, there is growing interest in helping countries respond to the challenge of noncommunicable disease, and expanded prequalification might make consolidated regional or global procurement an option.

When resources are scarce, the imperative to make good use of what is available increases. There is room to improve product safety and quality by making better use, where appropriate, of information already collected in the routine operations of government, business, and nonprofits. For regulatory agencies this means collecting, managing, and sharing data with their counterpart agencies abroad and with other interested parties. Donor funding could help minimize the technical obstacles and expense associated with this process, helping to tip the balance of tradeoffs in favor of greater openness.

Recommendation 3-3: Development partners, including multilateral and bilateral donors and private philanthropic organizations, should support countries and regional organizations in pursuing greater collaboration for regulating food and medical products. This collaboration can include harmonization and mutual recognition of data or standards, equivalence agreements, and regulatory reliance.

Data sharing produces a global public good; the information generated can inform public policy and risk analysis and can be used to answer valuable research questions. The technical cost of data sharing is an obstacle, and one that donors could help overcome. Providing data standards and a common platform could also help build trust among regulators and advance the long-term goal of regulatory harmonization.

The Role of Commerce

Regulatory enforcement can improve the products in a market, but the regulator's power to change manufacturing is limited if industry is not investing in quality. Investing in quality can grow business and improve efficiency, but such benefits are not always clear to people in a position to change business practices. Even when they are, if the capital available comes at too high a price, the manufacturer's calculations will not favor improvement. Development banks and bilateral development finance organizations can adjust this calculation, both with advisory services and with concessional financing (meaning loans with more generous terms than the market would offer).

Recommendation 3-4: Development finance institutions such as the United States International Development Finance Corporation, the

International Finance Corporation (IFC), the UK CDC Group, and the European development finance banks should create vehicles to finance producers, distributors, and retailers in low-and middle-income countries interested in meeting regulatory standards. This would involve advisory services and, when appropriate, concessional financing.

There are also global companies that are active in quality testing, but not necessarily expanding in low- and middle-income countries. Their products can be used in manufacturing, and are often helpful in downstream product monitoring, testing for authenticity or contamination at point of use, or at point of entry to a country. While such testing is not a substitute for regulatory checks or full quality assurance in manufacturing, it is important to the system.

There is a need for inexpensive, field-ready screening tools to detect product contamination or fraud in low- and middle-income countries. There is also a need to decrease the cost associated with existing technologies. When the market for such products is small the companies that make them do not have good reason to invest in manufacturing or build their distribution systems. The lack of both optimal manufacturing and distribution creates a vicious cycle where small markets lead to weak incentives to invest, which keep the market small.

Recommendation 3-5: The United States International Development Finance Corporation, the International Finance Corporation (IFC), the UK CDC Group, and the European development finance banks should provide advisory services and concessional financing to manufacturers of quality and safety screening technologies to optimize manufacturing and create stronger distribution systems in low- and middle-income countries.

Expanding the Evidence Base for Regulatory Policy

Regulatory science is not well studied, and the evidence base to support regulatory policy is lean, especially in small countries, regional consortia, and low- and middle-income countries. Advanced agencies have ways to collaborate with academia to advance the science they need; the FDA Centers of Excellence in Regulatory Science is a good example of such collaboration. These centers research priorities in the FDA's strategic plan; they are evaluated on how well the information they produce informs the agency's work and advances public health. This model of dedicated research centers run in collaboration with universities could be adapted globally.

Recommendation 3-6: The National Institutes of Health, in collaboration with the U.S. Food and Drug Administration and the U.S. Agency for International Development, should develop a network of Global Centers of Excellence in Regulatory Science for research and capacity building to identify and address the challenges of ensuring food and drug safety in low- and middle-income countries.

The proposed Centers of Excellence would be primarily research centers, distinguishing them from the similarly named Regional Centers of Regulatory Excellence in Africa, which are mainly concerned with training. In order to ensure that the research generated is useful and tailored to questions of local priority, the proposed centers would involve regulators in setting a research agenda. This type of demand-drive research would promote the implementation and uptake of research findings.

THE ROLE OF THE NATIONAL GOVERNMENT

Regulatory quality is one of the six aggregate measures of good governance the World Bank uses to assess the institutions in a country. Like other features of good governance, the capacity of the regulatory system is partly determined by the willingness of the national government to support it. Much of the regulatory agency's effectiveness, efficiency, and independence is determined by a country's political leaders, who are ultimately responsible for creating an environment conducive to product safety.

Legal Protections

Providing the legal framework for product safety may be the most fundamental step national political leaders can take to protect food and medical products in their countries. Legal provisions define which institutions are part of the regulatory system, the ways they are involved, and their ability to enforce rules. The process of drafting food and drug laws is complicated; it may be eased by consulting model legislation, though model laws often require significant modifications to the local context. In any case, the legal mandate for regulatory systems should give special attention to their independence, sustainable financing, and provisions for cooperation.

A lack of political interference in an agency's decisions and in the hiring and firing of technical staff is necessary for consumer confidence in the system. It also allows industry to function with confidence that the rules affecting their products will be applied in a predictable way. A regulatory agency's independence in partly dependent on a stable and diversified revenue stream, something that is difficult to ensure in low- and middle-income countries. Broadly speaking, governments have a short list of revenue sources from which to fund regulatory agencies: taxes, fees on industry, earmarks, or some combination thereof. There are administrative and economic tradeoffs associated with all options, and the appropriate balance of revenue should be revisited periodically.

Sustainable financing is important because all agencies are facing the limits of their resources. Sharing work with foreign agencies can allow countries to work more efficiently. International cooperation is so central to modern food and medical product regulation that the WHO and the FAO assess it in their regulatory benchmarking evaluations. Government support for this cooperation is essential, and the drafting or revision of national food and drug laws is an important time to ensure legislative provisions are in place.

Supporting the regulatory agency is part of government's responsibility to its citizens. Political leaders can take a meaningful step toward meeting that responsibility through attention to the laws that protect it.

Recommendation 4-1: National governments should guarantee in legislation that national regulatory agencies be independent and financially viable, with statutes that encourage cooperation with other agencies and require a scientific basis for decision making.

Regulatory resources should be allocated with an eye to those jobs that add the maximum value for effort. Political leaders should give regulators clear authority for international coordination and guidance on how to resolve any tension between national and shared international responsibilities.

THE ROLE OF THE REGULATORY AGENCY

Decision makers at the regulatory agency have the most direct, proximal control over the actions taken to mitigate product safety risks. Attention to risk and work sharing could increase the scientific rigor at regulatory agencies and ensure their resources are deployed efficiently.

Strategies for Controlling Risk

Decisions about how to reduce risks facing the regulatory agency are, even at the most advanced agencies, often made in the face of uncertainty. Therefore, an over-emphasis on the ideal quantitative risk analysis could be a barrier to progress in low- and middle-income countries. While acknowledging that the public sector is often limited in its data and analytic capacity, regulators can still use risk-based approaches to make use of the information they have. A risk-based framework, even when applied to imperfect data, draws attention to the relative vulnerabilities in a system.

A risk-based regulatory system protects health; it also has positive spillovers for the economy, but quantifying these effects is challenging. There is a time lag between a regulatory policy going into effect and measurable changes taking place. Cost-to-benefit analysis and analysis of the causal pathway between regulatory policy and health and welfare gains are useful in estimating the value of the agency's work. Such analyses depend on technical skills that are not always available, however. The proposed Centers of Excellence in Regulatory Science could undertake these assessments when necessary. Regulators can facilitate evaluation by clearly stating the goals of regulatory policies, the data that would be evaluated in an assessment, and sources for these data.

Regulatory work is highly technical and complicated and, when done properly, invisible to the consumer. This poses a barrier to public appreciation for the regulatory agency, but one that can be overcome with effective communication, data about the risks facing the consumer, and steps the agency is taking to mitigate them.

It can be difficult for regulators to advocate the importance of their work when things are going well. For this reason, agencies need a plan for crisis communication. The reason some crises undermine the agency and others cause people to rally behind it is not clear, but effective communication plays a role. Regulators should be prepared to communicate clearly and honestly during a crisis, because the tragedy of a product safety failure is only compounded if the agency fails to use the spotlight as an impetus for change.

Recommendation 5-1: National regulatory authorities should take a risk-based approach to the regulation of food and medicines. This includes:

- **a. Developing effective data systems to systematically identify areas of greatest risk;**
- **b. Participating in research, data sharing, technology adoption, and training activities with international partners;**
- **c. Growing capacity to assess the health and economic impacts of regulation, and using this information to inform actions to protect public health;**
- **d. Communicating about risks, including the uncertainty around them, especially during a crisis; and**
- **e. Communicating the ways regulation improves quality, safety, and access, using different strategies to convey this information to government leaders, regulated industry, and the public.**

The tools available to make regulators' work more efficient are best deployed to deal with the formal operations of known producers and distributors, but in low- and middle-income countries food and medical products are often sold outside these channels. In such circumstances, regulators may need to give more attention to strategies that drive consumer preference to the best feasible option and increase the reach of safe products.

Informal food markets account for an estimated 80 percent of food sold in low- and middle-income countries and are especially prominent sources of nutrient-dense, animal-source foods. Though storage and handling conditions are poor, shutting down informal markets is not usually logistically feasible and would have disastrous consequences for food security and livelihoods. Educational campaigns to help consumers mitigate the risks facing them can help, as can intervention at aggregating points on the supply chain (e.g., the slaughterhouse, dairy plant, or wholesale market).

Regulatory agencies may be more likely to consider aggressive enforcement as a way to combat the informal medicines market, though enforcement alone is unlikely to put informal sellers out of business. In low- and middle-income countries, the informal market is a response to a demand for medicines that exceeds the supply. Accreditation is one tool with promise to improve the reach of good-quality medical products; consumer education and mobile technology can also be effective.

Recommendation 5-2: National regulatory agencies should use evidence to guide strategies to reduce the risk posed by informal markets. Strategies to consider include accreditation or licensing to formalize sellers, consumer education, and increasing competition from regulated products.

Steps taken to mitigate the risks of informal markets can be expected to have disproportionate returns for the regulatory agency because they depend on local knowledge. The question remains as to how to manage work in a way that allows regulators to devote more time to these value-added activities. Jobs that do not pay off in terms of better understanding or control of local risks are best approached with an eye to making use of the work of other trusted authorities.

Cooperation and Delegation

Regulatory collaboration can result in more opportunities for training and exchange and a more predictable business environment. It also allows for more opportunities for networking with other experts, and can thereby improve the scientific rigor of regulatory decisions. Regional networks are one venue for regulatory cooperation, but regulators can also make unilateral decisions to rely on certain authorities' decisions. UN agencies also provide valuable tools; some private organizations produce useful technical guidelines. To serve the goal of maximizing staff time and effort, regulators should look for ways to make use of publicly available resources.

Recommendation 5-3: National regulatory authorities should take advantage of global tools to support regulatory actions. Resources from United Nations agencies, including World Health Organization prequalification and Codex standards, are examples of such tools, as are the third-party standards increasingly used in food and agriculture.

Realizing the benefits of work sharing requires identifying those tasks best shared among countries, as well as those best devolved to sub-national authorities. There is no universal blueprint to guide the coordination of multiple levels of government. Developing technical capacity at the local level and governance capacity (the skills that allow levels to work together) at all levels is important for effective delegation.

Recommendation 5-4: National regulatory authorities should determine which functions are most effectively and efficiently carried out directly by the agency and which can be delegated to state or local authorities; collaboration and data sharing among domestic agencies should be part of any delegation plan.

Efficient division of work, collaboration, and information sharing are tools that can help regulators manage the increasing challenge of protecting the safety of food and the quality of medical products in their countries. National governments and development partners also have roles to play to advance this goal. This report sets out a strategy for building regulatory systems in low- and middle-income countries; progress toward this end can be measured with regular benchmarking assessments.

1

Introduction

The U.S. Food and Drug Administration (FDA) was established more than a century ago in response to growing public concern with quack remedies, unhygienic food production, and the adulteration of food and medicines (FDA, 2018b). Commerce was also a driving force in the agency's creation; legitimate food and medicine producers found it difficult to comply with myriad conflicting standards promulgated by state authorities (FDA, 2018b). The agency continues to serve the same basic purpose today. A public health agency, the FDA sets a bar for a market of $2.5 trillion every year, accounting for 20 cents of every dollar the U.S. consumer spends (FDA, 2018a).

Over its history, the FDA has changed in response to various threats and crises. The sulfanilamide crisis of 1937 led to the 1938 Food, Drug and Cosmetic Act, which authorized premarket approval of drugs for safety (Sharfstein, 2018). The thalidomide scare led to the 1962 amendments that set standards for drug efficacy (Sharfstein, 2018). More recently, adulterated heparin made under unhygienic conditions in China caused hundreds of allergic reactions, some ending in death, in the United States (Pew Health Group, 2011). The crisis, occurring at the same time as well-publicized food safety scandals in China, brought to light liabilities in modern, multinational supply chains (Pew Health Group, 2011). (Some more recent product safety crises not otherwise mentioned in this report are shown in Table 1-1.)

The FDA's response included a reorganization, creating a deputy commissioner for Global Regulatory Operations and Policy (Alliance for a Stronger FDA, 2012). The agency also opened foreign offices, where the staff could work more closely with partners overseas (GAO, 2010). With

TABLE 1-1
Product Safety Crises Around the World

Incident	Country	Date of Incident or Publication	Source
Infant formula contaminated with melamine sickens almost 300,000 babies	China	2008	Xiu and Klein, 2010
More than 200 deaths and 1,000 hospitalizations from contaminated heart medication	Pakistan	2011	WHO, 2013
More than 3,800 cases and 54 deaths from Shiga-toxin on sprouts	Germany	2011	Frank et al., 2011
Over 750 people in 20 states contract fungal meningitis from contaminated steroid injections, resulting in 64 deaths	United States	2012	CDC, 2015
Between 4 and 16 percent of anti-tuberculosis drugs sampled from pharmacies fail quality testing	Angola, Brazil, China, DR Congo, Egypt, Ethiopia, Ghana, India, Kenya, Nigeria, Russia, Rwanda, Tanzania, Thailand, Turkey, Uganda, and Zambia	2013	Bate et al., 2013
Almost a third of emergency contraceptives fail quality testing	Peru	2014	Monge et al., 2014
Aflatoxicosis outbreak with 68 cases and 20 deaths	Tanzania	2016	Kamala et al., 2018
Between 72,000 and 169,000 child pneumonia deaths a year because of substandard and falsified antibiotics	Low- and middle-income countries	2017	Campbell and Theodoratou, 2017

Poor quality antimalarials cause between 8,500 and 19,800 deaths a year[a]	Sub-Saharan Africa	2017	Goodman and Yeung, 2017
1,060 people sickened and at least 216 killed in *listeria* outbreak	South Africa	2017–2018	Whitworth, 2018
Substandard vaccine for diphtheria, pertussis, and tetanus administered to between 215,000 and 615,000 children	China	2018	*The Lancet*, 2018
Cyclosporiasis linked to Fresh Express salad mix sold at McDonald's restaurants; 511 confirmed cases in 16 states	United States	2018	CDC, 2018
Contaminated formula causes 32 cases of *salmonella* in infants and young children	Belgium, France, and Luxembourg	2018–2019	European Center for Disease Prevention and Control and European Food Safety Authority, 2019
About 1,700 confirmed cases of cyclosporiasis in 33 states	United States	2019	CDC, 2018

[a] Based on WHO estimates of 435,000 malaria deaths a year, 93 percent in Africa (WHO, 2019).

increasing international involvement comes an increasing workload. FDA staff overseas influence product decisions affecting the U.S. consumer. More broadly, their job includes building capacity in their host countries, working with their counterparts in foreign governments and with industry and academic representatives (GAO, 2010).

The goal of capacity building was at the center of the agency's commission, in 2011, of a consensus study report from the Institute of Medicine (IOM). The committee's report, published in 2012, emphasized trade, work sharing, and training as tools to improve food and medical product safety in the United States and around the world (IOM, 2012). The report gave a strategy, discussed later in this chapter, for the FDA and other global health and development organizations to consider in their work, mostly limited to a 3- to 5-year action plan.

The world has changed since the 2012 release of *Ensuring Safe Foods and Medical Products Through Stronger Regulatory Systems Abroad*. The FDA has also changed, so has donor assistance for health in low- and middle-income countries. In light of these developments, the FDA asked the National Academies of Sciences, Engineering, and Medicine to convene a committee to revisit the topic of strengthening food and drug regulatory systems (hereafter, regulatory systems). Box 1-1 shows the task the agency gave the committee. More information about the committee members answering this charge can be found in Appendix A.

THE COMMITTEE'S APPROACH TO ITS CHARGE

The committee met four times; a delegation of committee members and staff also had a public meeting in San Jose, Costa Rica, the site of an FDA regional office. Agendas for public workshops are shown in Appendix B.[1] In closed session, the committee discussed the information presented at the public workshops in January, February, and April 2019. They also reviewed relevant literature as cited in this report. Members of the public submitted articles and written testimony for the committee's consideration, available upon request from the National Academies' Public Records Office (paro@nas.edu).

To better understand how emerging technologies can be used at regulatory agencies, the committee put out a call for comments. This call, shown in Appendix C, was published on the study webpage and shared with regulatory systems experts at the World Health Organization (WHO) and the Food and Agriculture Organization of the United Nations (FAO); it was

[1] Please note revisions to the listed agendas. For example, speakers from the FDA and the USAID were not able to attend the first meeting because of the federal government shutdown. The sponsor briefed the committee on its charge via a conference call on February 5, 2019.

BOX 1-1
Statement of Task

The 2012 Institute of Medicine report *Ensuring Safe Food and Medical Products Through Stronger Regulatory Systems Abroad* put considerable emphasis on capacity building in developing countries as a means to improve the safety of food and drugs around the world. Recommendations called for building regulatory agencies in low- and middle-income countries; strengthening the scientific and technical underpinning for regulatory policy and action; increasing technical support for post-market surveillance; and placing regulatory systems in the global economic, development, and trade agenda. While progress has been made on these goals, the global regulatory landscape has changed significantly since 2012. It is therefore timely to assess progress made towards these goals and the current regulatory landscape. With this in mind, an ad hoc committee convened by the National Academies of Sciences, Engineering, and Medicine should:

- Assess how the challenges and opportunities facing regulators have changed since 2012 and how technology and innovation affect their work;
- Discuss the transition off donor aid and the capacity of regulatory systems to ensure the safety and quality of regulated products, the lack of post-market surveillance in many countries, and the challenges of regulating the informal medicines market;
- Recommend ways to increase scientific robustness at food and drug regulatory agencies in low- and middle-income countries;
- Identify concrete steps to raise visibility and increase investment in global food and drug safety as part of global health, development, and trade programming of the United States government and internationally; and
- Examine the priority given to food and drug regulatory systems in low- and middle-income countries and suggest ways to increase will for developing such systems at the national or regional levels.

also advertised on the National Academies' social media, with the National Academies' global health and food and nutrition listservs, and through the committee members' networks. Responses to the call for information are included in the public access file for this project.

In its deliberations and during the sponsor orientation to the project, the committee clarified the intended audience for this report. The study sponsors at the FDA are a primary audience, as are other U.S. government agencies that work in the field, such as the U.S. Department of Agriculture (USDA) and the U.S. Agency for International Development (USAID), as well as global health organizations such as the WHO and the FAO, and the development banks. Producers of food and medical products are an audience for this report, both individually and through their trade groups, as are consumer organizations. Regulators in low- and middle-income countries are another audience for this report. More broadly, this document should be of interest to anyone with a stake in global health, development, or international affairs.

Discussions with the study sponsor also helped the committee set its analytic strategy, in recognition of the wide range of technical areas the Statement of Task introduces. Food safety and the safety and quality of medical products are clearly relevant but are dealt with broadly and positioned as they are relevant to trends in global health and development. Matters of governance and management are central to this report; these are topics that are important to regulators but are not necessarily the technical evaluation, compliance, or enforcement matters that command their attention day to day. This report does deal with some questions of special interest to regulators, such as the underpinning of a risk-based system and the challenges of informal markets, communication, and data management. Nevertheless, the balance of the material presented in this report is concerned with common principles related to both food and medicines regulation, and the relationship of the field to global health and development.

To this end, the report is not divided along interests of food, medicines, and other medical products, but is roughly organized against the Statement of Task shown in Box 1-1. This chapter deals with the 2012 report and with the changes affecting regulatory systems in the last 8 years. The next chapter gives an overview of the broader health and development context affecting demand for food and medicines and support for regulatory systems. It also introduces risk-based decision making and other key concepts in modern product safety, along with the main stakeholders and some of the relationships among them. Chapter 3 discusses how regulatory systems could be better incorporated into global health and development programming, highlighting the role of development finance and long-term investment in regulatory agencies, ways to expand the WHO prequalification program, and other strategies to advance regulatory science. Chapter 4 moves to the national level in considering a conducive environment for regulatory systems and the pros and cons of different organizational and financing strategies. Chapter 5 turns to internal matters at regulatory agencies, suggesting ways to improve scientific rigor and make work more manageable.

Core principles of regulation apply to both food and medical products. There are other similarities, such as a diverse set of manufacturers, the value of preventive controls, and the importance of surveillance. Because this report is concerned with regulatory systems and product safety, much of the discussion applies broadly to both sectors. For those points that apply to just one field, this is noted in the discussion.

This report recognizes the responsibility national regulators have for the products in their markets. At the same time, these agencies do not operate in a vacuum. With this in mind, the report gives considerable emphasis to actions at the global and national level that foster the ability of the regulatory agency to function. The recommendations start at the global level, then move to changes at the country level beyond those in the control of the regulatory agency or agencies. The last group of recommendations suggests actions at the level of regulatory agencies.

Understanding the committee's task also requires some attention to those topics that are outside the scope of this report. The problem of falsified and substandard medicines is not a primary focus of this report, insomuch as it is one of the challenges facing medicines regulators. Similarly, this report does not contain detailed analysis of trade policy or original data collection. While food safety is a topic of this report, the related topic of agricultural development is only tangentially relevant.

GLOBALIZATION AND REGULATORY SYSTEMS

The FDA Office of International Programs commissioned *Ensuring Safe Foods and Medical Products Through Stronger Regulatory Systems Abroad* at a time when several high-profile product safety lapses had called into question the extent to which the United States, or any country, could reasonably guarantee the safety of food and medicines produced and distributed through expansive global supply chains. The idea that food or medicines could be poisoned and the source never come to light scared the American public. But at the root of the heparin scandal was a more vexing, if mundane, problem: The agency charged with regulating global supply chains did not have the authority or the resources to work outside of the United States (Senak, 2008).

Food and medical products are produced outside the United States because globalization changed the way companies do business. It changed government too, though perhaps more slowly. In 2012, the U.S. Department of Health and Human Services released its first ever global strategy, a document that highlighted how the health of Americans was intertwined with the health of people around the world (HHS, 2012; Sullivan, 2018). Securing supply chains was a main objective of this strategy, which cited risk analysis and strengthening of partnerships with other regulatory agencies as essential means to product safety (HHS, 2012). Across all its goals, the strategy emphasized how improving the health of Americans requires working outside of the United States, and also working outside of what would typically be seen as health, on economic and infrastructure problems sometimes at the root of disease and early death (Daulaire, 2012; HHS, 2012).

The 2012 Report Recommendations

This position was consistent with the strategy outlined in the 2012 report on regulatory systems. The Statement of Task for the report, shown with its recommendations in Appendix D, asked the committee to identify core elements of regulatory systems and priority areas for FDA engagement, with special consideration given to certain emerging markets. As Appendix D shows the report's recommendations were divided into domestic and international actions; it also sets out the committee's assessment of the main gaps in regulatory systems in developing countries, and its summary of the essential elements of regulatory systems. In its advice to the FDA and other U.S. organizations, the committee encouraged the agency to make risk the guiding principle for all the agency's operations. The committee recognized that the most pressing risks facing the agency may be in foreign producers, and that the FDA's authorizing legislation might need to be changed if it were to redirect substantial attention abroad (thereby assuring the safety of ingredients and products imported to the United States). Considering the challenges of monitoring products and tracking disease in developing countries, the report also recommended that various U.S. government agencies give more support to surveillance systems in low- and middle-income countries, both post-market surveillance for medicines and foodborne disease surveillance (through the PulseNet program, for example).

As Appendix D shows, several of the 2012 report's recommendations dealt with securing multinational supply chains. The report also recognized that, while globalization of supply chains had caused some of the problems facing the agency, it also held the promise to solve them (IOM, 2012). For example, the scale of foreign manufacturing exceeds the reach of the FDA's inspectorate, but the sharing of inspection reports from other advanced regulatory agencies can help close the gap. The committee encouraged the agency to move to paperless systems to improve efficiency and to facilitate work sharing among other advanced regulatory agencies, and recommended sharing of inspection reports as a goal for both governments and industry associations.

Similarly, global trade and telecommunications have made the world more connected. In response, governments of both developed and emerging economies have, since 1999, come together in the G20, an economic forum that aims to promote international financial stability (Ramachandran, 2015). The 2012 report identified the G20 as the ideal venue to promote the importance of strengthening regulatory systems. It also explored ways the private sector and academia might be better included in the discussion about food and drug safety. In an effort to direct private sector and academic research at developing technologies suitable for use in low- and middle-income countries, the report suggested that the FDA and the USDA implement Cooperative Research and Development Agreements for fraud detection, tracking, and verification technologies. It also suggested ways for regulatory agencies in developing countries to draw on the technical depth in their countries' private industries and universities.

One of the main messages in the 2012 report concerned the training and retention of quality staff in the regulatory agencies. The committee stressed the value of training for regulators in low- and middle-income countries, as a means both to improve the regulatory process and to build professionalism and morale at agencies. To this end, it recommended that the FDA invest in training for staff at its counterpart agencies overseas (IOM, 2012).

Investing in safe food and good-quality medical products abroad is one of the best examples of development assistance being in the enlightened self-interest of the donor. Around and after the release of the 2012 report on strengthening regulatory systems, more donor and international organizations took an interest in a previously neglected piece of health systems. Without overstating the relationship between the 2012 report and subsequent developments, a brief review of progress in the field is necessary.

Major Changes in the Field

The last 10 years have seen increasing recognition of the interconnectedness of regulatory systems, meaning that regulatory failures in one market can have consequences somewhere else. This recognition, combined with an increased demand for medical products and safe foods (discussed in the next chapter), has spurred interest in strengthening regulatory systems. It is important to note that this interest has been a gradual evolution. Even when considering progress since the previous report, an observer might raise the valid observation that the root problems are largely the same today as they were in 2012. Factors such as weak institutions or limited technical capacity are, though improving, still relevant underlying conditions.

Key programs may have discrete start times, but they are representative of a broader change happening slowly. Nevertheless, some orientation to important changes since 2012 is necessary to understand the field today. Given its role as the global standard setting body in health, and its work with governments around the world on health and health systems, the WHO has had a role in many of these efforts (WHO, n.d.-c).

Efforts to Build Medical Products Systems

One of the most prominent examples of the WHO's involvement in regulatory systems is in action against falsified and substandard medicines. In 2012, WHO member states passed a resolution against falsified and substandard medicines[2] (WHO, 2017a, n.d.-b). The immediate work plan under this mechanism included strengthening national regulatory authorities and quality control labs, and collaborating on surveillance and monitoring of the drug supply (WHO, 2012). To this end, the WHO launched a global surveillance and monitoring system for unsafe medicines in 2013 (WHO, 2017c, n.d.-a). Part of the system includes training regulators, including inspectors, quality control technicians, and experts in surveillance and enforcement (WHO, n.d.-a). Reporting suspect medicines to central authorities in Geneva via electronic rapid alert is also an important part of the process (WHO, n.d.-a). Regulators can then check their reports against a secure international database of compromised products and work with WHO staff to determine if the same problem is showing up in multiple markets (WHO, n.d.-a).

Global coordination on falsified and substandard medicines has exponentially grown the muscle of regulatory agencies in low- and middle-income countries. Through central reporting, places that once had little to no capacity to monitor markets now have information from around the world at their fingertips, making it easier to identify global patterns. Almost 1,500 falsified or substandard products were reported to the WHO between 2013 and 2017 (WHO, 2017c). The first report from the Global Surveillance and Monitoring team acknowledged that finding problems depends more than anything on active market surveillance, as well as on staff at the national regulatory authority reporting the problems to the central WHO team. Even so, their data suggest that inexpensive, lifesaving medicines—anti-malarials, antibiotics, and painkillers (including anesthetics)—are commonly compromised (WHO, 2017b).

Earlier research on the problem of falsified and substandard medicines commented on the irony of the problem: that the very data that would compel greater attention to medicines regulatory systems are unavailable when the systems do not work (Buckley et al., 2013; IOM, 2013). The WHO programing on falsified and substandard medicines has improved the situation. With more attention directed to identifying poor quality medicines in the market, donors and governments have better reason to invest in fighting them. Two years after the World Health Assembly's first resolution against falsified and substandard medicines, it passed another resolution on

[2] The resolution referred to "substandard, spurious, falsely-labelled, falsified, counterfeit" medicines, a descriptor used at the time, and since rejected in favor of the clearer "falsified and substandard."

strengthening regulatory systems, urging member states to invest in their regulatory systems, to pool resources for essential jobs when necessary, and to take stock of the strengths and weaknesses in their systems so to create useful institutional development plans (WHO, 2014). The resolution also affirmed support for the WHO to evaluate the performance of regulatory systems, something discussed in more detail in Chapter 3 (WHO, 2014).

Whether the 2014 WHO resolution, with its emphasis on pooling resources, was the cause or an effect of greater interest in regulatory co-operation internationally cannot be said, but international harmonization of regulatory requirements has improved considerably in the last 5 years. For example, the International Council for Harmonisation of Technical Requirements for Pharmaceuticals for Human Use (ICH), a group that brings together medicines regulators, industry associations, and other stakeholders to facilitate harmonization, has grown considerably in the last 5 years. At its founding in 1990, the ICH included the regulatory authorities of the European Commission, Japan, and the United States, and three associations representing innovator pharmaceutical companies (ICH, n.d.-a). Ten years later, ICH members included those countries that conduct new molecule review, representing about 15 percent of the world's population (WHO, 2002). Today, in addition to the three founding members, ICH members and observers include over 20 countries and 6 regional harmonization groups, as well as an expanding list of industry associations and other organizations involved in regulatory policy or procurement, or otherwise affected by regulatory harmonization (ICH, 2018). New observers in the ICH include the East African Community, the Southern African Development Community, and the Pan American Network of Drug Regulatory Authorities (ICH, 2018). The changing, more global composition of the ICH allows medicines regulators in small or low-income countries to have a say in the harmonization process, including the consensus building process for new guidelines, and to build valuable relationships with their counterparts in foreign agencies (ICH, n.d.-b).

Harmonization for medical device regulation has a shorter history; the medical device group analogous to the ICH, the International Medical Device Regulators Forum, was founded in 2011 to promote regulatory convergence for devices (IMDRF, n.d.-b). The forum involves regulatory authorities from nine countries and the European Union, as well the WHO and several regional affiliates (IMDRF, n.d.-a). In an effort to reduce the regulatory burden on both device manufactures and industry, members developed a single audit system that would meet requirements of all participating regulators (FDA, 2019b). The FDA and other regulatory agencies, including those of China, Brazil, and Russia, now accept these audit reports, allowing them to perform far fewer inspections (FDA, 2019b).

Other venues for regulatory collaboration stem directly from the WHO's interest in the topic. Since 2012, the International Coalition of Medicines Regulatory Authorities has brought together the heads of agencies for strategic discussions about common problems (ICMRA, 2017a,c). Twenty-four regulatory agencies are members; the shared priorities identified at coalition meetings give some insight into the challenges facing them, including crisis management, pharmacovigilance, and supply chain integrity (ICMRA, 2017b).

Efforts to Build Food Safety Systems

Food safety is also the subject of growing international interest. In 2015, the WHO released the results of an 8-year investigation on the global burden of foodborne disease (WHO, 2015a). While acknowledging serious limitations in the data, mostly because of problems with surveillance and laboratory capacity, the report estimated 600 million cases of foodborne illness in 2010, causing over 400,000 deaths (WHO, 2015a). Children under 5, though accounting for only about 9 percent of the world's population, accounted for almost a third of these deaths, or 125,000 a year (WHO, 2015a,b).

It is hard to overstate the importance of the WHO report and the work of the Foodborne Disease Burden Epidemiology Reference Group. It has been long accepted that foodborne disease is underreported, and even when it is reported, the source of the infection is often difficult to pinpoint (Bettencourt, 2010). The WHO report, for the first time, put numeric parameters on the scope of the problem. As the report explained, foodborne disease, which is most common in the world's poorest countries, can impair people's ability to work, thereby aggravating the cycle of poverty (WHO, 2015a). When magnified over the population, this pattern holds back economic development and also damages local industries dependent on safe food, such as tourism (WHO, 2015a). Agriculture, a field that employs almost 60 percent of the work force in the least developed countries, and about a third in all low- and middle-income ones, stands to be particularly hurt (World Bank, 2019).

At the same time, there are limitations to the WHO report that influence countries' ability to respond to it. Despite citing goals of improving assessment and response to foodborne illness at the national level, results from the study were published in regional aggregates, partly because of methodological limitations in the way the data were derived (Havelaar, 2016; Havelaar et al., 2015; WHO, 2015a). This means that no country can reference its results to monitor its performance over time or relative to other countries, and no regulatory agency can use the results to advocate for increased investment in food safety.

Another challenge in controlling foodborne outbreaks has always been identifying the contaminated food and knowing when the pathogen entered the supply chain. A powerful tool to answer these questions came on the market in the late 2000s, when the cost and time needed for genome sequencing fell dramatically (Stevens et al., 2017). By sequencing the genomes of pathogens drawn from a restaurant, processing plant, or farm and comparing patient samples, it is possible to identify the source of an outbreak quickly, making it easier to remove the source from the food supply before more people get sick. Such is the idea behind GenomeTrakr, a program the FDA started in 2012 (Timme et al., 2018). The program brings together different food safety laboratories, including those at the FDA field offices, state and local health departments, and universities, to sequence the genomes of pathogens from patients and environmental sources (restaurants, farms, etc.) (Timme et al., 2018). The laboratories then report the sequences to a public database. Labs around the world can participate in GenomeTrakr, allowing for international outbreak investigation and identification of relationships between geographically disparate samples, something necessary in a global food supply chain (FDA, 2019a).

But the promise of whole genome technology remains out of reach for many countries. All of the 20 GenomeTrakr labs outside the United States are in high-income countries. The laboratory analysis necessary to support genome sequencing is often unavailable in developing countries, where more routine testing for chemical and biological hazards is challenging (Vipham et al., 2018). Other equipment and consumables needed to run a modern food laboratory can be prohibitively expensive or hard to find, and their use depends on human capacity for laboratory analysis, another major limitation (FAO, n.d.; Vipham et al., 2018).

Building capacity for food safety is a focus of the Food Safety Modernization Act (FDA, 2013). Passed in 2011, this law shifted the FDA's emphasis from reaction to prevention so, as then deputy commissioner for Foods Michael Taylor described it, "prudent preventive measures will be systematically built into all parts of the food system" (Taylor, 2011). For example, under the act, food companies are required to identify the points in processing when contamination is most likely, and put preventive measures in place at those steps (Olson, 2011). This emphasis on prevention is part of a global trend in food regulation, moving away from a "strict policing function of government," and involving greater partnership with the private sector (Jaffee et al., 2019).

Globalization of the food supply was a key impetus for the Food Safety Modernization Act, which put requirements on food importers to guarantee that foreign producers they work with meet the requirements for the U.S. market (Olson, 2011). To this end, it formalized recognition of third-party accreditation, allowing producers with certain recognized certifications[3] improved access to U.S. markets (FDA, 2018c). It also mandated more frequent inspections of producers abroad. Increasing inspections puts greater demand on the FDA, although the budget necessary to support such inspections has not been forthcoming (Olson, 2011). The agency's Food Safety Dashboard posts information about the private sector's compliance with the new requirements (FDA, n.d.).

Work Sharing and Capacity Building

The increase in inspections required of the FDA is a function of the increased complexity of modern manufacturing systems. In an effort to adapt to these changes and simultaneously improve efficiency, the agency has recently entered into agreements to allow the agency to recognize the procedures, especially the inspections, of European authorities (FDA, 2017a). Mutual recognition agreements allow the United States and its counterpart European agencies to avoid duplicating work and to spend their inspection resources more efficiently (FDA, 2018d). The mutual recognition agreements currently in force with the FDA pertain to inspections of medicine and biologics producers, as well as organizations conducting clinical trials (EMA, n.d.). A recent National Academies committee concluded that, given the complex, global nature of modern drug supply chains, work sharing with other regulatory authorities is an essential part of modern good regulatory practice (NASEM, 2020).

The movement to greater collaboration among regulatory agencies allows the participating agencies to work more efficiently. By reducing duplication, it also eases the regulatory burden on industry. By making market entry fairer and more predictable for all firms, it facilitates trade. But maximizing the return on regulatory collaboration depends on the agency's ability to employ and retain competent staff, a problem discussed at length in the 2012 report (IOM, 2012).

As part of the implementation of the aforementioned report, the FDA worked with the International Food Protection Training Institute, the Regulatory Affairs Professional Society, and the WHO to articulate the necessary skills for government regulatory jobs in low- and middle-income countries (PAHO, 2016; Preston et al., 2013). Figure 1-1 shows the framework developed, highlighting the basic skills regulators need to work well, skills that align with ongoing WHO benchmarking reviews discussed at length in Chapter 3 (PAHO, 2016).

---

[3] To date, the American National Standards Institute, the American National Standards Institute–ASQ National Accreditation Board, and International Accreditation Services, Inc., are the only recognized accreditation bodies (FDA, 2019a).

The Need for More Progress

The last 5 years have been a time of advancement for regulatory systems, characterized by growing technical capacity, especially in middle-income countries, and increased global cooperation on problems such as falsified and substandard medicines and foodborne disease control. Some of the leadership has come from obvious stakeholders such as the FDA, the European Union regulatory authorities, and the ICH. It is encouraging to note that a broader cross-section of organizations is taking an interest in the topic; the WHO, the FAO, development banks, and bilateral donors are investing in regulatory systems, as are international donors such as Gavi[4] and Global Fund.[5] Such progress is encouraging for anyone in global health or health systems.

At the same time, there is still considerable work to be done. In Africa, for example, all but one country has a medicines regulatory agency, though only seven of these agencies have the legal mandate for essential regulatory functions (Ndomondo-Sigonda et al., 2017; WHO, 2010). This means that even some basic medicines regulatory jobs such as market authorization, inspection, and quality control are neglected in a part of the world with serious health needs and demand for medical products. The situation is no better in many larger countries. In India, which produces 20 percent of the world's generic medicines, core responsibilities are shared among several federal and state-level agencies, so standards for even basic functions such as licensing can vary widely (Gupta et al., 2017). Medicines registration, perhaps the most basic responsibility of the regulatory agency, is also a problem in China; at its peak in 2015 the registration backlog was about 22,000 applications (Xu et al., 2018).

The state of food regulatory systems is often much less clear. This is partly because evaluations of the sort cited in the previous paragraph, taking stock of the food safety systems across countries, do not exist for most developing countries, and evaluations that have been done are not often publicly available (Jaffee et al., 2019). The evidence suggests, however, that the cost of unsafe food to the domestic economy in low- and middle-income countries is 15 to 20 times higher than the estimated costs of forgone trade (Jaffee et al., 2019). Furthermore, as the recent World Bank report explained, the gaps between a population's needs and the existing food safety infrastructure tend to depend most on the country's development level, with the greatest need in lower-middle-income countries, particularly the large ones (Jaffee et al., 2019). Across developing countries, it is especially difficult to design food safety systems that reach the poorest people.

[4] Officially, Gavi, the Vaccine Alliance.

[5] Officially, the Global Fund to Fight AIDS, Tuberculosis and Malaria.

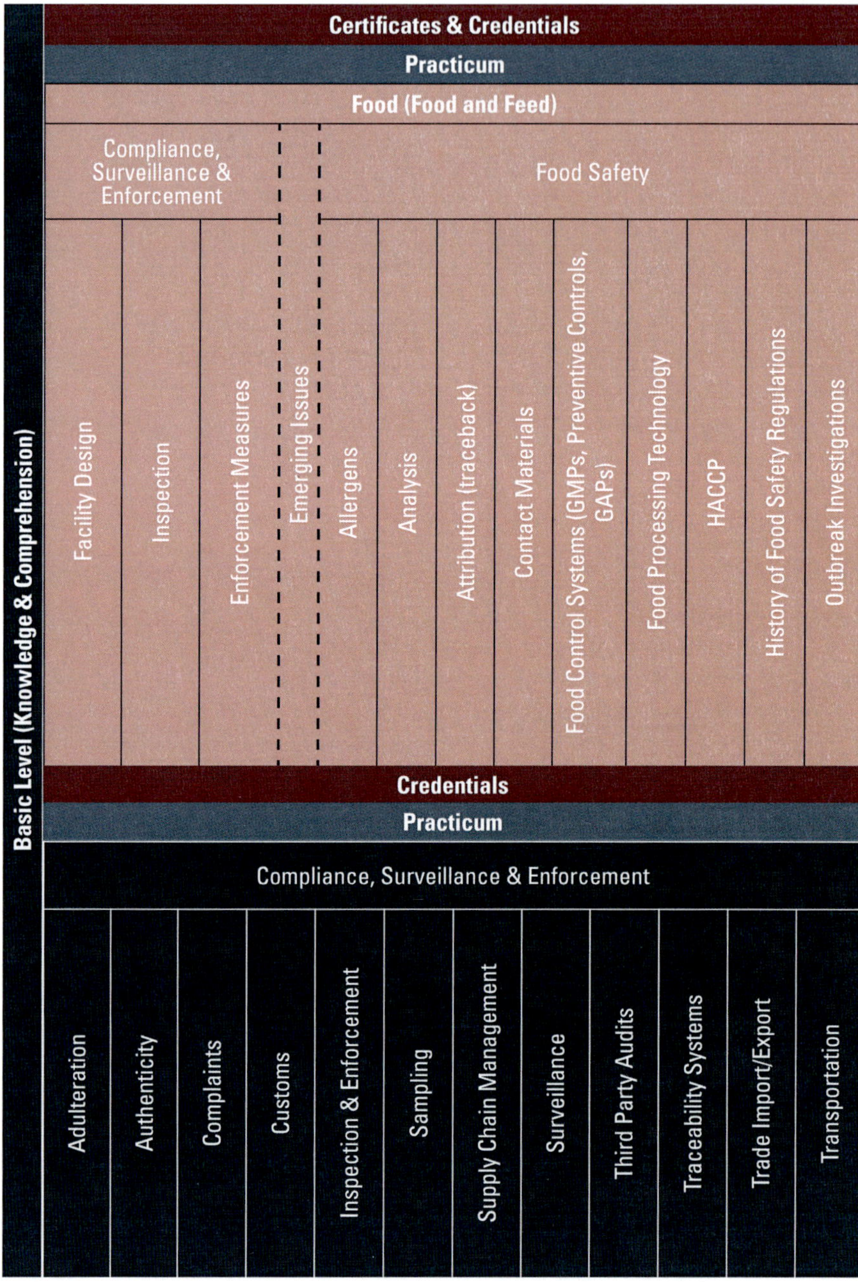

FIGURE 1-1 Global food and medical product basic curriculum framework for food, feed, or medical product regulatory functions.
SOURCE: IFPTI, 2015.

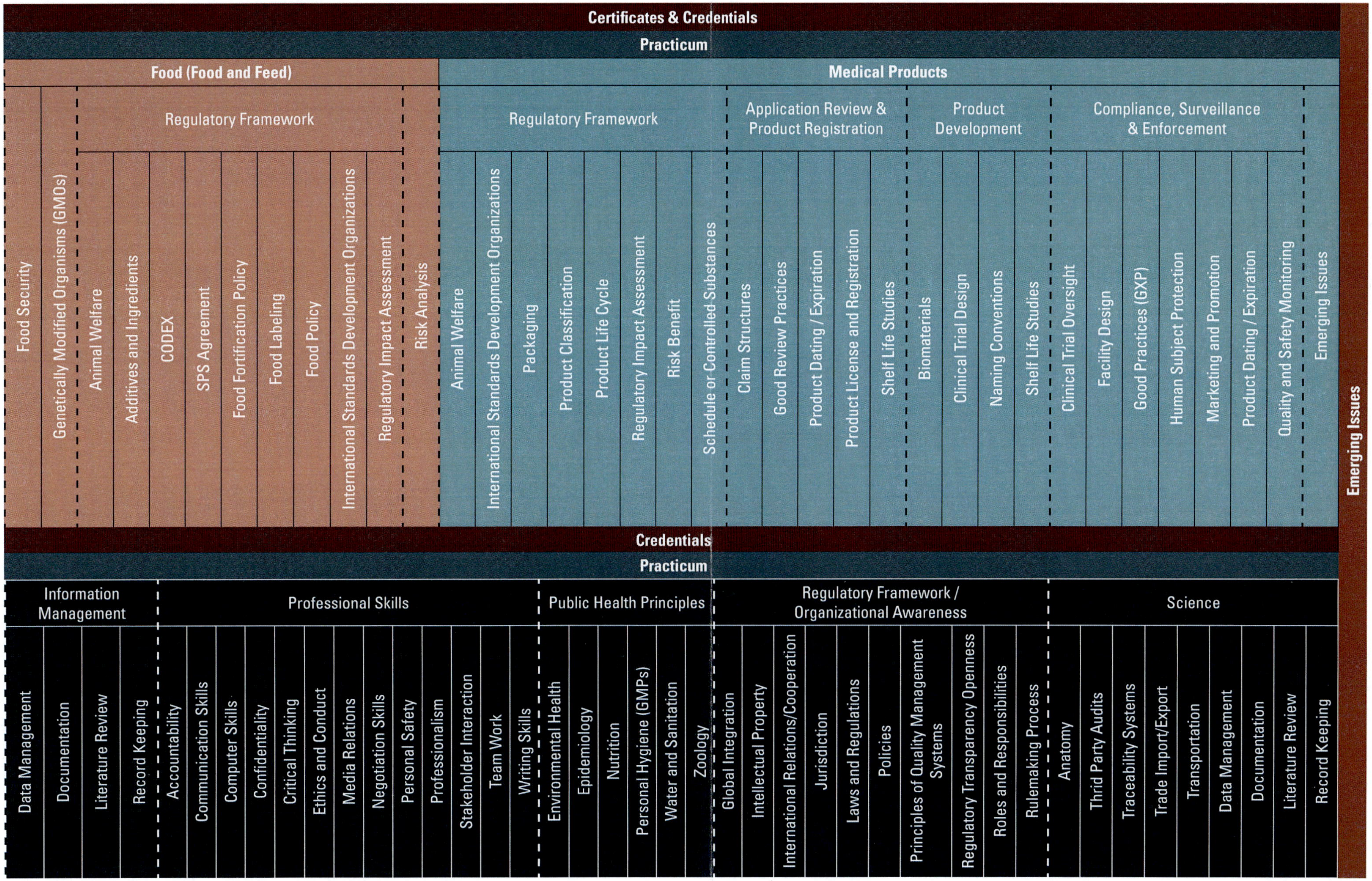
Certificates & Credentials
Practicum
Food (Food and Feed)
Food Security
Genetically Modified Organisms (GMOs)
Regulatory Framework
Animal Welfare
Additives and Ingredients
CODEX
SPS Agreement
Food Fortification Policy
Food Labeling
Food Policy
International Standards Development Organizations
Regulatory Impact Assessment
Risk Analysis
Medical Products
Regulatory Framework
Animal Welfare
International Standards Development Organizations
Packaging
Product Classification
Product Life Cycle
Regulatory Impact Assessment
Risk Benefit
Schedule or Controlled Substances
Application Review & Product Registration
Claim Structures
Good Review Practices
Product Dating / Expiration
Product License and Registration
Shelf Life Studies
Product Development
Biomaterials
Clinical Trial Design
Naming Conventions
Shelf Life Studies
Compliance, Surveillance & Enforcement
Clinical Trial Oversight
Facility Design
Good Practices (GXP)
Human Subject Protection
Marketing and Promotion
Product Dating / Expiration
Quality and Safety Monitoring
Emerging Issues
Emerging Issues
Credentials
Practicum
Information Management
Data Management
Documentation
Literature Review
Record Keeping
Professional Skills
Accountability
Communication Skills
Computer Skills
Confidentiality
Critical Thinking
Ethics and Conduct
Media Relations
Negotiation Skills
Personal Safety
Professionalism
Stakeholder Interaction
Team Work
Writing Skills
Public Health Principles
Environmental Health
Epidemiology
Nutrition
Personal Hygiene (GMPs)
Water and Sanitation
Zoology
Regulatory Framework / Organizational Awareness
Global Integration
Intellectual Property
International Relations/Cooperation
Jurisdiction
Laws and Regulations
Policies
Principles of Quality Management Systems
Regulatory Transparency Openness
Roles and Responsibilities
Rulemaking Process
Science
Anatomy
Thrid Party Audits
Traceability Systems
Trade Import/Export
Transportation
Data Management
Documentation
Literature Review
Record Keeping

Subsistence farmers have little choice regarding their water source, animal bedding, or crop inputs; traditional markets are, almost by definition, not operating to modern hygiene standards. An increased emphasis on meeting international standards in certain market segments can also do unintended harm to the most vulnerable, when food that fails to meet standards for export or chain-market retail is then redirected to places the poorest people shop (Jaffee et al., 2019).

Keeping Pace with Innovative Technology

It is not surprising that countries with fewer resources and weaker institutions have problems with regulatory systems. Even the most advanced agencies are facing the limits of what they can reasonably accomplish. Part of the challenge is that new technologies strain regulatory systems that were designed for conceptually simpler products (Califf et al., 2019). The regulatory approvals process for biosimilars, the generic equivalents of large-molecule, biologically active medicines, is one example of this challenge. Complex biologic medicines, used increasingly since the early 2000s, work in the immune system in novel ways, complicating comparisons between the innovator and biosimilar products (Falit et al., 2015). The regulatory review process for small-molecule generics is therefore not entirely transferable to biosimilars, but an unnecessarily onerous process creates a barrier to market entry, thereby limiting access, driving up costs, and encouraging confusion among prescribers (Falit et al., 2015). The health of many people, and millions of dollars, depend on getting the regulatory framework right.

The computer algorithms used to support health also present regulatory challenges. Mobile apps, for example, might claim to diagnose melanomas at an early stage; internet genetic counseling might offer genome interpretation for a fee. Such technology has vast potential to improve health, and an equally vast potential for quackery (JASON, 2017). It is not yet clear what revisions to the regulatory review process for such technologies might best protect public health without impeding scientific progress. Even if staff time were not a rate-limiting step in the review process, artificial intelligence has forced regulators to confront the Collingridge dilemma: the problem of understanding how to make policies that govern technology when the technology is still developing (Genus and Stirling, 2018). By acting too soon, regulators risk taking actions that hold back science, in this case by forcing artificial intelligence into an unsuitable review process but, by waiting too long, they miss the window to act, let snake oil salesmen prosper, or both.

Gene therapy is another field unfolding faster than the policy to regulate it. Gene editing technology, and the gene drivers that can spread a trait in wild populations, have great potential in health and agriculture and could be used to eliminate dengue or malaria from mosquitoes, for example

(Dooley, 2018). It can be difficult to balance this potential against ecological concerns, especially given uncertainty about how modified genes might spread in the wild (Dooley, 2018).

Other technologies challenge quality assurance systems. In the last few years, regulators in the United States and Europe have grappled with enforcement of good manufacturing practices when devices are made on 3D printers, and with ensuring the safety of robotic devices in a way that controls the risk to patients and still encourages creativity on the part of industry (Califf et al., 2019; FDA, 2017b; Leenes et al., 2017).

All these questions require new and different kinds of skills among regulators (Slikker et al., 2018). And, as the 2012 report made clear, recruiting and retaining staff who understand novel technology to the regulatory agency is difficult; government cannot offer the same salaries as the private sector, and prospective employees may fear losing skills by taking work that removes them, even briefly, from the technological frontlines (IOM, 2012).

As the regulatory agencies in developed countries confront the limits of their processes, it is timely to consider ways these systems might be adapted to today's markets. In places where the regulatory infrastructure is new or, in the case of medical devices, sometimes nonexistent, there is an opportunity to design a system with the benefit of hindsight. One option is to change laws to allow recognition of foreign review or registration, or to allow for work sharing with neighboring countries. Changing legislation may be a slow process, however, and politicians may balk at any ceding of sovereignty, real or perceived. When the process is designed with an emphasis on efficiency, that calculation can change.

This report sets out a cross-cutting strategy to support good-quality, wholesome food, and quality, safe, effective medical products around the world. The goal of this report is to build on the momentum for strengthening regulatory systems developing over the last 10 years and to set a course for continued progress.

REFERENCES

Alliance for a Stronger FDA. 2012. *The FDA as a global actor: A summary report.* https://strengthenfda.org/2012/10/02/the-fda-as-a-global-actor-a-summary-report (accessed April 29, 2019).

Bate, R., P. Jensen, K. Hess, L. Mooney, and J. Milligan. 2013. Substandard and falsified anti-tuberculosis drugs: A preliminary field analysis. *International Journal of Tuberculosis and Lung Disease* 17(3):308–311.

Bettencourt, L. A. 2010. *A complex mystery: Finding the sources of foodborne disease outbreaks.* https://www.foodsafety.gov/blog/complexmystery.html (accessed May 9, 2019).

Buckley, G., J. Riviere, and L. O. Gostin. 2013. What to do about unsafe medicines? *BMJ* 347:f5064.

Califf, R. M., M. Hamburg, J. E. Henney, D. A. Kessler, M. McClellan, A. C. von Eschenbach, and F. Young. 2019. Seven former FDA commissioners: The FDA should be an independent federal agency. *Health Affairs 38*(1):84–86.

Campbell, H., and E. Theodoratou. 2017. Childhood pneumonia. In *A study on the public health and socioeconomic impact of substandard and falsified medical products*. Geneva, Switzerland: World Health Organization.

CDC (U.S. Centers for Disease Control and Prevention). 2015. *Multistate outbreak of fungal meningitis and other infections*. https://www.cdc.gov/hai/outbreaks/meningitis.html (accessed November 11, 2019).

CDC. 2018. *Multistate outbreak of cyclosporiasis linked to Fresh Express salad mix sold at McDonald's restaurants—United States, 2018: Final update*. https://www.cdc.gov/parasites/cyclosporiasis/outbreaks/2018/b-071318/index.html (accessed October 3, 2019).

Daulaire, N. 2012. The global health strategy of the Department of Health and Human Services: Building on the lessons of PEPFAR. *Health Affairs (Millwood)* 31(7):1573–1577.

Dooley, C. 2018. Regulatory silos: Assessing the United States' regulation of biotechnology in the age of gene drives. *Georgetown International Environmental Law Review* 30:547–568.

EMA (European Medicines Agency). n.d. *United States*. https://www.ema.europa.eu/en/partners-networks/international-activities/bilateral-interactions-non-eu-regulators/united-states (accessed May 3, 2019).

European Centre for Disease Prevention and Control and European Food Safety Authority. 2019. *Multi-country outbreak of* Salmonella *Poona infections linked to consumption of infant formula*. Stockholm, Sweden: European Centre for Disease Prevention and Control.

Falit, B. P., S. C. Singh, and T. A. Brennan. 2015. Biosimilar competition in the United States: Statutory incentives, payers, and pharmacy benefit managers. *Health Affairs (Millwood)* 34(2):294–301.

FAO (Food and Agricultural Organization of the United Nations). n.d. *Strengthening laboratory services*. http://www.fao.org/fileadmin/user_upload/agns/pdf/factsheets/StrengtheningLaboratoryServices.pdf (accessed October 4, 2019).

FDA (U.S. Food and Drug Administration). 2013. *FDA's international food safety capacity-building plan: Food Safety Modernization Act 305*. Washington, DC: HHS, FDA.

FDA. 2017a. *Frequently asked questions/The mutual recognition agreement*. https://www.fda.gov/media/103391/download (accessed May 3, 2019).

FDA. 2017b. *Technical considerations for additive manufactured medical devices*. https://www.fda.gov/media/97633/download (accessed May 9, 2019).

FDA. 2018a. *Fact sheet: FDA at a glance*. https://www.fda.gov/about-fda/fda-basics/fact-sheet-fda-glance (accessed April 29, 2019).

FDA. 2018b. *FDA's evolving regulatory powers*. https://www.fda.gov/about-fda/history-fdas-internal-organization/fdas-evolving-regulatory-powers (accessed April 29, 2019).

FDA. 2018c. *FSMA final rule on accredited third-party certification*. https://www.fda.gov/food/food-safety-modernization-act-fsma/fsma-final-rule-accredited-third-party-certification (accessed Septmeber 9, 2019).

FDA. 2018d. *Mutual recognition agreement (MRA)*. https://www.fda.gov/international-programs/international-arrangements/mutual-recognition-agreement-mra (accessed May 3, 2019).

FDA. 2019a. *Accredited third-party certification program: Public registry of accredited third-party certification bodies*. https://www.fda.gov/food/importing-food-products-united-states/accredited-third-party-certification-program-public-registry-accredited-third-party-certification (accessed October 3, 2019).

FDA. 2019b. *GenomeTrakr fast facts*. https://www.fda.gov/food/whole-genome-sequencing-wgs-program/genometrakr-fast-facts (accessed May 3, 2019).

FDA. n.d. *FDA data dashboard.* https://datadashboard.fda.gov/ora/index.htm (accessed October 3, 2019).

Frank, C., D. Werber, J. P. Cramer, M. Askar, M. Faber, M. an der Heiden, H. Bernard, A. Fruth, R. Prager, A. Spode, M. Wadl, A. Zoufaly, S. Jordan, M. J. Kemper, P. Follin, L. Müller, L. A. King, B. Rosner, U. Buchholz, K. Stark, and G. Krause. 2011. Epidemic profile of shiga-toxin–producing *Escherichia coli* o104:H4 outbreak in Germany. *New England Journal of Medicine* 365(19):1771–1780.

GAO (U.S. Government Accountability Office). 2010. *Food and Drug Administration: Overseas offices have taken steps to help ensure import safety, but more long-term planning is needed.* GAO 10-960: Report to the Committee on Oversight and Government Reform, House of Representatives September 2010.

Genus, A., and A. Stirling. 2018. Collingridge and the dilemma of control: Towards responsible and accountable innovation. *Research Policy* 47(1):61–69.

Goodman, S., and S. Yeung. 2017. Malaria in sub-Saharan Africa. In *A study on the public health and socioeconomic impact of substandard and falsified medical products.* Geneva, Switzerland: World Health Organization.

Gupta, M., M. Shridhar, G. N. Singh, and A. Khadem. 2017. Regulatory systems in India: An important global hub for medical products and technologies. *WHO Drug Information* 31(3).

Havelaar, A. 2016. *The global burden of foodborne disease: Overview and implications.* https://www.rivm.nl/sites/default/files/2018-11/Prof%20Havelaar.pdf (accessed December 10, 2019).

Havelaar, A., M. D. Kirk, P. R. Torgerson, H. J. Gibb, T. Hald, R. J. Lake, et al. 2015. World Health Organization global estimates and regional comparisons of the burden of foodborne disease in 2010. *PLoS Medicine* 12(12):e1001923.

HHS (U.S. Department of Health and Human Services). 2012. *The global strategy of the U.S. Department of Health and Human Services.* https://www.hhs.gov/sites/default/files/hhs-global-strategy.pdf (accessed April 29, 2019).

ICH (International Council for Harmonisation of Technical Requirements for Pharmaceuticals for Human Use). 2018. *Current members and observers.* https://www.ich.org/about/members-observers.html (accessed April 29, 2019).

ICH. n.d.-a. *History.* https://www.ich.org/about/history.html (accessed April 29, 2019).

ICH. n.d.-b. *Value of membership.* https://www.ich.org/about/value-of-membership.html (accessed April 29, 2019).

ICMRA (International Coalition of Medicines Regulatory Authorities). 2017a. *History of ICMRA.* http://icmra.info/drupal/history (accessed May 3, 2019).

ICMRA. 2017b. *ICMRA membership country/region and regulatory authority's website.* http://www.icmra.info/drupal/participatingRegulatoryAuthorities (accessed April 29, 2019).

ICMRA. 2017c. *International coalition of medicines regulatory authorities (ICMRA).* http://www.icmra.info/drupal/en (accessed April 29, 2019).

IFPTI (International Food Protection Training Institute). 2015. *Global food and medical product framework.* http://ifpti.org/wp-content/uploads/2017/03/FINAL-GLOBAL-CURRICULUM-FRAMEWORK.pdf (accessed May 9, 2019).

IMDRF (International Medical Device Regulators Forum). n.d.-a. *About IMDRF* http://www.imdrf.org/about/about.asp (accessed May 3, 2019).

IMDRF. n.d.-b. *International Medical Device Regulators Forum.* http://www.imdrf.org (accessed April 29, 2019).

IOM (Institute of Medicine). 2012. *Ensuring safe foods and medical products through stronger regulatory systems abroad.* Washington, DC: The National Academies Press.

IOM. 2013. *Countering the problem of falsified and substandard drugs.* Washington, DC: The National Academies Press.

Jaffee, S., S. Henson, L. Unnevehr, D. Grace, and E. Cassou. 2019. *The safe food imperative: Accelerating progress in low- and middle-income countries.* Agriculture and food series. Washington, DC: The World Bank.

JASON. 2017. *Artificial intelligence for health and health care.* McClean, VA: The MITRE Corporation.

Kamala, A., C. Shirima, B. Jani, M. Bakari, H. Sillo, N. Rusibamayila, S. De Saeger, M. Kimanya, Y. Y. Gong, and A. Simba. 2018. Outbreak of an acute aflatoxicosis in Tanzania during 2016. *World Mycotoxin Journal* 11(3):311–320.

Leenes, R., E. Palmerini, B.-J. Koops, A. Bertolini, P. Salvini, and F. Lucivero. 2017. Regulatory challenges of robotics: Some guidelines for addressing legal and ethical issues. *Law, Innovation and Technology* 1–44.

Monge, M. E., P. Dwivedi, M. Zhou, M. Payne, C. Harris, B. House, Y. Juggins, P. Cizmarik, P. N. Newton, F. M. Fernandez, and D. Jenkins. 2014. A tiered analytical approach for investigating poor-quality emergency contraceptives. *PLoS One* 9(4):e95353.

NASEM (National Academies of Sciences, Engineering, and Medicine). 2020. *Regulating medicines in a globalized world: The need for increased reliance among regulators.* Washington, DC: The National Academies Press.

Ndomondo-Sigonda, M., J. Miot, S. Naidoo, A. Dodoo, and E. Kaale. 2017. Medicines regulation in Africa: Current state and opportunities. *Society of Pharmaceutical Medicine* 31(6):383–397.

Olson, E. D. 2011. Protecting food safety: More needs to be done to keep pace with scientific advances and the changing food supply. *Health Affairs (Millwood)* 30(5):915–923.

PAHO (Pan American Health Organization). 2016. *Global regulatory curriculum—A joint effort.* Paper read at VIII Conference of the Pan American Network on Drugs Regulatory Harmonization, October 19–21, 2016, Mexico City.

Pew Health Group. 2011. *After heparin: Protecting consumers from the risks of substandard and counterfeit drugs.* Washington, DC: Pew Health Group.

Preston, C., S. Azatyan, T. Bell, K. Bond, J. Bradsher, M. Brumfield, G. Buckley, T. Hughes, S. Kane, S. Keramidas, M. Miller, M. Morrison, L. Rago, J. Riviere, M. L. Valdez, and G. Wojtala. 2013. *Developing a global curriculum for regulators.* Washington, DC: National Academy of Medicine.

Ramachandran, J. 2015. *G20 finance ministers committed to sustainable development.* http://www.ipsnews.net/2015/09/g20-finance-ministers-committed-to-sustainable-development (accessed May 9, 2019).

Senak, M. 2008. Heparin at the center of the storm. *American Health & Drug Benefits* 1(6):23–24.

Sharfstein, J. M. 2018. *The public health crisis survival guide: Leadership and management in trying times.* New York: Oxford University Press.

Slikker, W., Jr., T. A. de Souza Lima, D. Archella, J. B. J. de Silva, T. Barton-Maclaren, L. Bo, D. Buvinich, Q. Chaudhry, P. Chuan, H. Deluyker, G. Domselaar, M. Freitas, B. Hardy, H. G. Eichler, M. Hugas, K. Lee, C. D. Liao, L. H. Loo, H. Okuda, O. E. Orisakwe, A. Patri, C. Sactitono, L. Shi, P. Silva, F. Sistare, S. Thakkar, W. Tong, M. L. Valdez, M. Whelan, and A. Zhao-Wong. 2018. Emerging technologies for food and drug safety. *Regulatory Toxicology Pharmacology* 98:115–128.

Stevens, E. L., R. Timme, E. W. Brown, M. W. Allard, E. Strain, K. Bunning, and S. Musser. 2017. The public health impact of a publically available, environmental database of microbial genomes. *Frontiers in Microbiology* 8:808.

Sullivan, T. 2018. *HHS global health strategy 2012*. https://www.policymed.com/2012/03/hhs-global-health-strategy-2012.html (accessed May 9, 2019).

Taylor, M. R. 2011. Will the Food Safety Modernization Act help prevent outbreaks of foodborne illness? *New England Journal of Medicine* 365(9):e18.

The Lancet. 2018. Vaccine scandal and confidence crisis in China. *The Lancet* 392(10145):360.

Timme, R. E., H. Rand, M. Sanchez Leon, M. Hoffmann, E. Strain, M. Allard, D. Roberson, and J. D. Baugher. 2018. GenomeTrakr proficiency testing for foodborne pathogen surveillance: An exercise from 2015. *Microbial Genomics* 4(7):e000185.

Vipham, J. L., B. D. Chaves, and V. Trinetta. 2018. Mind the gaps: How can food safety gaps be addressed in developing nations? *Animal Frontiers* 8(4):16–25.

Whitworth, J. 2018. *Experts say consumers must demand improved food safety in Africa*. https://www.foodsafetynews.com/2018/09/experts-say-consumers-must-demand-improved-food-safety-in-africa (accessed July 25, 2019).

WHO (World Health Organization). 2002. *The impact of implementation of ICH guidelines in non-ICH countries*. Geneva, Switzerland: World Health Organization.

WHO. 2010. *Assessment of medicines regulatory systems in Sub-Saharan African countries: An overview of findings from 26 assessment reports*. Geneva, Switzerland: World Health Organization.

WHO. 2012. *WHA65.19 Substandard/spurious/falsely-labelled/falsified/counterfeit medical products*. https://www.who.int/medicines/regulation/ssffc/mechanism/WHA65.19_English.pdf (accessed April 29, 2019).

WHO. 2013. *Deadly medicines contamination in Pakistan*. https://www.who.int/features/2013/pakistan_medicine_safety/en (accessed September 20, 2019).

WHO. 2014. *Regulatory system strengthening for medical products*. http://apps.who.int/medicinedocs/documents/s21456en/s21456en.pdf (accessed April 29, 2019).

WHO. 2015a. *WHO estimates of the global burden of foodborne diseases: Foodborne disease burden epidemiology reference group 2007–2015*. Geneva, Switzerland: World Health Organization.

WHO. 2015b. *WHO's first ever global estimates of foodborne diseases find children under 5 account for almost one third of deaths*. https://www.who.int/news-room/detail/03-12-2015-who-s-first-ever-global-estimates-of-foodborne-diseases-find-children-under-5-account-for-almost-one-third-of-deaths (accessed May 3, 2019).

WHO. 2017a. *Review of the member state mechanism on substandard/spurious/falselylabelled/falsified/counterfeit medical products*. Geneva, Switzerland: World Health Organization.

WHO. 2017b. *A study on the public health and socioeconomic impact of substandard and falsified medical products*. Geneva, Switzerland: World Health Organization.

WHO. 2017c. *WHO global surveillance and monitoring system for substandard and falsified medical products*. Geneva, Switzerland: World Health Organization.

WHO. 2019. *Malaria*. https://www.who.int/news-room/fact-sheets/detail/malaria (accessed November 18, 2019).

WHO. n.d.-a. *WHO global surveillance and monitoring system*. https://www.who.int/medicines/regulation/ssffc/surveillance/en (accessed December 23, 2019).

WHO. n.d.-b. *WHO role*. https://www.who.int/medicines/regulation/ssffc/role/en (accessed April 29, 2019).

WHO. n.d.-c. *Working for better health for everyone, everywhere*. https://www.who.int/about/what-we-do/who-brochure (accessed April 29, 2019).

World Bank. 2019. *Employment in agriculture (% of total employment) (modeled ILO estimate)*. https://data.worldbank.org/indicator/sl.agr.empl.zs?end=2018&name_desc=false&start=1991&view=map (accessed May 3, 2019).

Xiu, C., and K. K. Klein. 2010. Melamine in milk products in China: Examining the factors that led to deliberate use of the contaminant. *Food Policy* 35(5):463–470.

Xu, L., H. Gao, K. I. Kaitin, and L. Shao. 2018. Reforming China's drug regulatory system. *Nature Reviews: Drug Discovery* 17(12):858–859.

2

Regulatory Systems, Global Health, and Development

In 1998 the World Health Organization (WHO) first set out a list of essential public health functions, jobs that governments undertake to protect and promote health. These functions have been revisited over the years by different countries and organizations (WHO, 2018a). The various iterations share a common emphasis on health legislation, surveillance, governance, and financing and often on public health regulation and enforcement (WHO, 2018a). Box 2-1 shows one influential iteration of essential public health functions. It should be noted that these essential jobs produce what are described as *public goods*, meaning that they are both non-excludable (one person's consumption does not prevent others from consuming it) and non-rival (one person's consumption does not affect the amount left) (Moon et al., 2017). In general, tax money pays for public goods, making provision of these services difficult when the tax base is small and the needs are great.

Attention to public health and public goods in low- and middle-income countries has been a defining characteristic of the past 20 years, as indicated by the United Nations' (UN's) Sustainable Development Goals, and the previous set of international development targets, the Millennium Development Goals (UN, 2015, 2018b). The 2018 World Bank report *The Safe Food Imperative* pointed out the necessity of food safety for achieving at least seven of the Sustainable Development Goals, especially the goals of ending poverty, ending hunger, and promoting good health (Jaffee et al., 2019). Safe and quality medicines are equally essential for the first three Sustainable Development Goals. Indeed, a functioning regulatory system is related to most of the goals, sometimes indirectly, as a precursor to a

BOX 2-1
Essential Public Health Functions

- Monitoring, evaluation, and analysis of health status
- Public health surveillance, research, and control of risks and threats to health
- Health promotion
- Social participation in health
- Development of policies and institutional capacity for planning and management
- Strengthening of institutional capacity for regulation and enforcement
- Evaluation and promotion of equitable access to necessary health services
- Human resources development and training in public health
- Quality assurance in personal and population-based health services
- Research
- Mitigating the health consequences of emergencies and disasters

SOURCE: PAHO, 2002.

target, or as an outcome of progress in an area. Table 2-1 discusses these relationships.

Although the Sustainable Development Goals, like the Millennium Development Goals before them, emphasize health, they are broader than any one sector. Among the 169 unique targets for the 17 goals, one in particular has commanded an attention eclipsing almost anything else in global health today. Universal health coverage, mentioned as a target under the goal of promoting good health, has been described by Margaret Chan, former director general of the WHO, as "a beacon of hope for a healthier world" and "the most powerful concept that public health has to offer" (Chan, 2015; Chan and Brundtland, 2016; WHO, 2020). Universal coverage was endorsed by the UN General Assembly in 2012 (UN, 2012). Since then, it has been the subject of an ongoing World Bank and World Health Organization collaboration for monitoring (WHO and World Bank, 2015, 2017). Subsequent UN General Assemblies have reaffirmed and supported universal coverage, both as a part of the Sustainable Development Goals and independently; creating, for example, a Universal Health Coverage Day in 2017, and convening a meeting on the topic for heads of state and policy makers in September 2019 (UHC2030, 2019; UN, 2018a). The latter meeting produced a political declaration wherein countries committed to increasing availability of quality, effective medicines, and adequate, healthy food (UN, 2019a). The recent political declaration was also notable for its mention of "the importance of strengthening regulatory and legislative frameworks" conducive to universal coverage (UN, 2019a).

Part of the appeal of universal coverage as a guiding principle for health is its promise to both improve quality of life and pull people out of poverty. Neglect of preventive services can lead to more serious conditions that are more expensive to treat; unhealthy people are not productive workers, and they have less energy to devote to their families, thereby limiting the potential of the next generation (Frenk and de Ferranti, 2012). Much of the discussion about universal coverage has emphasized the role of catastrophic health expenses in pushing people into poverty (Wagstaff et al., 2018a,b). Policy discussion has been similarly weighted to strategies for pooling funding and improving primary care (Lagomarsino et al., 2012; Moreno-Serra and Smith, 2012; Sachs, 2012). Even the indicators the UN expert working group developed to track progress toward universal coverage, indicators later endorsed by the UN Statistical Commission and the Economic and Social Council, track only measures of health service coverage (e.g., the percentage of health centers screening eligible women for cervical cancer) and financial protection (e.g., the percentage of households reporting catastrophic health expenses) (UHC2030, 2018; UN, 2019b).

Given this context, it is easy to miss the fact that universal coverage, as described in the Sustainable Development Goals, "include[s] financial risk protection, access to quality essential health-care services and *access to safe, effective, quality and affordable essential medicines and vaccines for all*" (emphasis added) (UN, 2016). In this definition, quality of medical products is given equal billing with essential services and financial protection, an attention that has not carried over to the policy discussion.

Part of the problem is that monitoring progress depends as much on the likelihood of reliable and straightforward measurement as on construct validity, and measurement has its own challenges (Dunning, 2016). There was much debate on the choice of services used to compute a valid proxy index for access to essential services (Hogan et al., 2018; Schensul, 2016; WHO and World Bank, 2017). Although nobody would deny the role of the regulatory system in reaching universal coverage, the concepts are harder to measure and therefore less amenable to direct, reliable data collection. A recent World Bank report expressed similar reservations regarding the indicators used to measure food safety systems (Jaffee et al., 2019). The 2017 *Lancet* Commission on Essential Medicines suggested indicators for the performance of regulatory systems including annual publication of risk-based quality surveys, publication of inspection reports, the proportion of manufacturers in a country using international good manufacturing practices, and the presence of a continuously updated agency website (Wirtz et al., 2017).

TABLE 2-1
Relationships Between Regulatory Systems and the Sustainable Development Goals

SDG	Relevant Targets	Direct or Indirect	Description
1 NO POVERTY	Targets emphasize social protection, access to basic public services and appropriate new technology.	Direct	Safe foods and quality medicines are an essential social protection. Ineffective or unsafe medicines and contaminated food cause illness and disability, which in turn impair children's capacity to learn, and adults' ability to work. Access to new technologies is also relevant to this topic; the introduction and control of medical devices and other health technologies are generally in the purview of the drug regulatory agency, though few low- or middle-income countries have regulatory provisions for device safety and performance.
2 ZERO HUNGER	Targets reflect concern with both productivity and market access among small-scale farmers. Other targets call out the role of international cooperation on agricultural research and extension, and the optimal functioning of national and international agriculture markets.	Direct	Food security requires access to safe foods; there is no food secuirty if the food supply is largely unsafe. Market access is related to the ability to meet safety standards, which can pose special challenges for small-scale farmers; cooperation and extension programs can improve productivity and safety, thereby reducing the burden of foodborne disease.
3 GOOD HEALTH AND WELL-BEING	Targets under this goal include universal coverage and reducing deaths from certain causes: maternal, neonatal, and child deaths; deaths from HIV, tuberculosis, or malaria; and premature death from noncommunicable diseases.	Direct	Safe, effective, quality-assured medical products are the cornerstone of a functional health system. Reducing the burden of noncommunicable disease is partly a function of having a safe and wholesome diet.

4 QUALITY EDUCATION	The quality and availability of higher education are targets, as is ensuring technical, engineering, and scientific skills in the workforce, and the skills that qualify people for employment and running businesses.	Indirect	Jobs in the food and pharmaceutical industries and in food and medicines regulation all require scientific and technical education at the secondary or tertiary level. Deficiencies in technical training were a common gap in the regulatory system, identified in the 2012 report; they persist today.
6 CLEAN WATER AND SANITATION	Targets call out sustainable water use and the problems caused by dumping and hazardous chemicals in the water supply.	Indirect	The suitability of the water supply for agricultural use is a frequent point of collaboration between food and agricultural and environmental agencies. Agricultural use of contaminated water is a common cause of foodborne illness.
8 DECENT WORK AND ECONOMIC GROWTH	Improving economic growth is at the center of this goal. Targets refer to the technological upgrading of industries that create jobs and produce valuable products, bringing more small- and medium-sized producers into the formal economy, and increasing foreign aid for trade.	Direct	Agriculture and medicines formulation are major employers in low- and middle-income countries. For want of investment in these industries, including technological investment, product quality suffers. The regulatory system can make it possible to grow these industries.

continued

TABLE 2-1 Continued

SDG	Relevant Targets	Direct or Indirect	Description
9 INDUSTRY, INNOVATION AND INFRASTRUCTURE	The first target refers to the regional and international infrastructure that supports economic development and human welfare. Targets mention the ability of small enterprises to participate in the formal economy, increasing scientific research and technical infrastructure in developing countries.	Indirect	Small agricultural producers account for a relatively large market share in low- and middle-income countries, and domestic drug formulation is often done by small and medium-sized businesses. These producers need capital and technical training to meet international standards, new technologies to reduce risk, and a strong testing and distribution infrastructure. A strong regulatory system can encourage competition and innovation, especially when rules are harmonized internationally.
10 REDUCED INEQUALITIES	This goal is concerned with, among other things, the use of World Trade Organization agreements to promote development. There are also financial ramifications to Codex standards, making the meaningful participation of developing country representatives in that international forum related to this goal.	Direct	The 2012 report emphasized trade as a tool to raise the floor on food quality in low- and middle-income countries; it also discussed problems with meaningful participation in Codex as a common gap in the food safety system. Inequitable access to quality food and safe medicines impedes social mobility and is a cause of inequality.
11 SUSTAINABLE CITIES AND COMMUNITIES	A target under this goal calls for a reduction in both deaths and the economic toll of disasters.	Direct	In humanitarian emergencies, access to safe food, vaccines, and medicines reduces loss of life.

12 RESPONSIBLE CONSUMPTION AND PRODUCTION	Among the targets for responsible consumption are the reduction of food waste all along the supply chain and capacity building among producers in developing countries.	Indirect	The 2012 report discussed the problems of food waste in developing countries, where it is generally between farm and market. Scientific and technical support to producers of food and medical products can help meet responsible production goals.
16 PEACE, JUSTICE AND STRONG INSTITUTIONS	This goal stresses the development of effective and transparent institutions as well as reduction in corruption and bribery.	Direct	Ensuring quality and safe food and medicines is an essential role of government; the regulatory agency's responsibility for public health also has economic ramifications, discussed in this report. A predictable, transparent, and functional regulatory agency provides society with public service, promotes fair competition and economic growth, and corrects market asymmetries.
17 PARTNERSHIPS FOR THE GOALS	Targets to advance partnerships emphasize the importance of dialogue between the public and private sectors and the need to marshal more money for sustainable development from multiple sources. The role of donor countries to honor development commitments is mentioned, as are building capacity in science and technology, increasing exports, and removing trade barriers in developing countries.	Indirect	The 2012 report suggested trade, particularly the access to lucrative markets in North America, Europe, and Japan, as the incentive needed to raise the floor on product quality in developing countries. While market access is an incentive for some producers, poverty creates markets for inferior products. Enforcement of relevant product safety regulations can improve quality in these markets; greater investment in development can offset the cost of doing so.

SOURCES: Eze et al., 2019; IOM, 2012; OECD, n.d.; UN, 2018b.

CONTINUING PROGRESS IN HEALTH AND DEVELOPMENT

Food and pharmaceutical systems are complicated, but the essential need for safe food and medicines is not. Current trends in global health and development (beyond the Sustainable Development Goals and universal coverage) make attention to the matter of regulatory systems all the more important.

Progress in Health

The last 20 years have seen major health improvement in low- and middle-income countries, with some of the most dramatic gains in children. Between 1990 and 2017, child mortality fell by more than 50 percent, in the least developed countries by over 60 percent (United Nations Inter-agency Group for Child Mortality Estimation, 2018). Neonatal mortality, which accounts for the largest share of child deaths, decreased by half between 1990 and 2017 (Hug et al., 2019). Stunting, a failure to grow reflective of both poor diet and frequent infection in early childhood, is also falling. In an analysis of population surveys from 36 low- and middle-income countries, almost 80 percent found a lower proportion of stunted children in 2012 than in 1990 (Tzioumis et al., 2016).

Similar progress has been made against common infectious diseases. By WHO estimates the treatment for tuberculosis patients averted about 54 million deaths between 2000 and 2017 (WHO, 2018b). The Global Burden of Disease study found HIV and AIDS deaths to be in decline, estimating 19 million years of life saved between 1996 and 2013, 70 percent of them in low- and middle-income countries, a success almost entirely attributable to the HIV medicines donors such as PEPFAR[1] and the Global Fund have provided (Murray et al., 2014). Even malaria, a disease that is difficult to treat, especially among pregnant women and young children, the latter accounting for the majority of malaria deaths, has fallen dramatically (Baird, 2013; Cibulskis et al., 2016; Global Burden of Disease Pediatrics Collaboration, 2016; Murray et al., 2014). By 2016 estimates, 1.2 billion cases of malaria were averted between 2001 and 2015, partly attributable to the use of insecticide-treated nets, residual indoor spraying for mosquitoes, and treatment with artemisinin combination therapy (Cibulskis et al., 2016). Encouraging trends can also be seen in vaccine-preventable diseases. The global program to eradicate polio, after floundering in the early 2000s, made important gains in the early 2010s, culminating in the global eradication of wild poliovirus type 2 in 2015 (Chan, 2017). The following year,

[1] Officially, The U.S. President's Emergency Plan for AIDS Relief.

indigenous measles was eliminated from the Americas (PAHO and WHO, 2016).

Donor organizations, including governments, multilateral organizations, and private philanthropy, deserve a great deal of credit for the health gains of the last 25 years. Maintaining these gains depends heavily on the workforce and infrastructure that support the delivery of health services. A 2014 Institute of Medicine (IOM) report concluded that support for health systems protects donors' multibillion-dollar investment in programs to fight HIV, tuberculosis, and malaria, and can help reduce dependence on foreign aid, which is changing rapidly in both manner and substance (IOM, 2014).

Global Development and Changes in Donor Assistance

Donor aid today may come from more sources than it once did but in smaller amounts, increasing the burden of managing the money in the recipient country (*The Economist*, 2015, 2016). There are also different strategies for distributing aid, including cash transfers, or payments made directly to the intended beneficiary (in the case of children, to their parents) or to governments for meeting certain targets (*The Economist*, 2015).

Aid for agriculture has varied over time, increasing sharply in times of global food crisis, as in 2008, and declining during times when other sectors were higher donor priorities (Cohen, 2015). Furthermore, aid to agriculture is often aimed at raising productivity, increasing the profitably of exports, and trade facilitation, making it difficult to disentangle what portion of aid for agriculture or rural development is intended primarily for food safety (ODI, 2012). A recent report on food safety in Africa found that of 518 projects donors funded between 2010 and 2017, the majority were aimed at improving market access for exports to both regional and global markets, with little to no attention given to matters of public health significance to Africans, such as reducing foodborne illness, improving surveillance, consumer education, research on local hazards, or practices in informal markets (GFSP, 2019).

Aid for health, after increasing sharply between 1990 and 2010, has leveled (Dieleman et al., 2016b; Moon and Omole, 2017). The Millennium Development Goals, with their relative emphasis on health, especially child mortality and major infectious diseases, drove much of the early increase in health spending (Dieleman et al., 2016b). As the Sustainable Development Goals, with their longer list of targets, become the motivators for global progress, it is possible that health could lose its relative prominence to donors. Even if it does not, the proportional weight of the donor contribution for health in the recipient countries is changing.

While external assistance makes up about a third of health spending[2] in low-income countries, it is far less, between 0.2 and 3.3 percent of health spending, in the middle-income countries that account for three-quarters of the world's population (Moon and Omole, 2017). The best strategy for foreign aid in middle-income countries, which are often both recipients of assistance and, through the UN system, donors, is debatable (Ottersen et al., 2017). Investments in the institutions that protect and improve health, including the workforce, management, service delivery, monitoring and surveillance, and essential medical products, may be the best use of donor funds in such circumstances (IOM, 2014). Attention to health systems is also seen as a remedy to a historical problem of "excessive emphasis on vertical programs devoted to control specific diseases and ... little attention to health systems as a whole" (Frenk et al., 2014).

The burden of disease is also changing in low- and middle-income countries, where malnutrition, infection, and maternal and child deaths are no longer the only, or even the main problems (Frenk et al., 2014). By Global Burden of Disease study estimates, almost three-quarters of all the world's deaths in 2016 were from noncommunicable diseases (*The Lancet*, 2017). High blood pressure and smoking are now the leading risk factors for early death and disability around the world (Institute for Health Metrics and Evaluation, 2017). Poor diet, especially one high in sodium or low in whole grains, fruits, and nuts, caused between 10 and 12 million deaths in 2017 alone (Afshin et al., 2019).

Changes in global patterns of disease and disability are in some way a result of a welcome increase in prosperity. In 2015, the percentage of the world population living in extreme poverty[3] fell below 10 percent, while the middle class[4] grew to over 3 billion (Kharas, 2017; World Bank, n.d.). The world is approaching a historic milestone: Around 2020 the majority of the world's population will live in a middle-class household (Kharas, 2017). Members of the middle class live longer, eat better, and use more health services than the poor; they are better educated and have more to invest in the education of their children. There is little to no evidence, however, that public services in much of the world are keeping pace with this change (Kharas, 2017).

Safe food and good-quality medical products are a necessary precursor to improved global health and development. No progress could have

[2] This estimate comes from the Institute for Health Metrics and Evaluation and does not include spending on food aid, food security, disaster relief, or water sanitation (Dieleman et al., 2016a).

[3] Extreme poverty is defined as living on less than $1.90 a day adjusted for purchasing power parity (World Bank, 2015).

[4] Defined by a household income between $10 and $100 a day, adjusted for purchasing power parity (Kharas, 2017).

been made against smallpox, for example, without an effective vaccine; well-nourished children are better able to survive infections and succeed in school. A growing demand for diverse foods and medicines is also a consequence of development. Recent projections show global demand for food increasing 74 percent by 2050 (Valin et al., 2014). The market for medical products is also changing. Drugs and vaccines for tropical diseases, for example, were once of little interest to pharmaceutical companies. In 2017, industry spent over $500 million, about 22 percent of total investment in these diseases, on research and product development (Chapman et al., 2018; WHO, 2019a). Research institutes in Brazil, India, Kenya, and Malaysia now develop new treatments for diseases of immense local importance (WHO, 2017).

Enthusiasm for such changes may be tempered by the realization that commensurate improvements in the institutions that guarantee the safety of food, improve the productivity of farmers, oversee the production of medicines, and test the quality of products on the market have not been forthcoming. It is difficult to even say how much donor aid has gone to strengthening regulatory systems, because this is not a category that is explicitly tracked. To understand the importance of the regulatory system to public health, it is necessary to first clarify the responsibilities of regulatory agencies, the conceptual underpinnings of the systems, and the roles of different stakeholders.

UNDERSTANDING THE REGULATORY PROCESS

The regulation of food and medicines is meant to correct a problem known as information asymmetry, a market failure where buyer and seller have unequal information about the products for sale. A carton of milk that has been contaminated looks identical to one treated hygienically; a vial of water and one of vaccine would be indistinguishable to even a sophisticated consumer. Sellers have little interest to correct market failures because such action would not be in any one player's market interest (Fagotto, 2013; Narrod et al., 2019). When consumers have incomplete information about safety, they cannot effectively choose safe products and reject unsafe ones. As a result, market incentives for safety are weak, requiring government regulatory action to balance the scales.

Box 2-2 lists the essential responsibilities of the regulatory agency as relates to medical products; Box 2-3 lists the same for foods. As these boxes indicate, there are differences in the regulation of foods and medicines. Food producers can usually enter the market without an external assessment of their product's safety, while market approval for medicines requires industry to demonstrate safety and effectiveness. At the same time, there are

BOX 2-2
Principal Regulatory Functions for Medical Products

- Licensing of the manufacture, import, export, distribution, promotion, and advertising of medicines
- Assessing the safety, efficacy, and quality of medicines, and issuing marketing authorization for individual products
- Inspecting and surveillance of manufacturers, importers, wholesalers, and dispensers of medicines
- Controlling and monitoring the quality of medicines on the market
- Controlling promotion and advertising of medicines
- Monitoring safety of marketed medicines, including collecting and analyzing adverse reaction reports
- Providing independent information on medicines to professionals and the public

SOURCES: Rägo and Santoso, 2008; WHO, 2003.

BOX 2-3
Principal Regulatory Functions for Foods

- Managing the national food control system, setting standards for safety, and implementing the national food control site
- Developing an emergency response procedure
- Inspecting manufacturers and suppliers, both their premises and processes, including importers or exporters when necessary, and issuing, revoking, or suspending market permits when necessary
- Participating in international food control activities
- Sampling food during harvest, processing, storage, transport, and sale to establish compliance, identify offenders, and collect data for risk-based decision making
- Conducting physical, microbial, and chemical analysis, the results of which can be used to determine compliance with standards
- Ensuring the food safety laboratories operate with accuracy, reliability, and repeatability of results
- Integrating with the public health system to ensure reliable intelligence on the incidence of foodborne disease and its relationship to food contamination
- Identifying food unfit for consumption or food deceptively sold, and taking remedial action
- Providing stakeholders from farm to table with independent, unbiased information about food safety

SOURCE: Adapted from FAO, 2003.

many similarities, especially the shared responsibility for quality assurance, inspection, and enforcement of laws.

There is also a broad conceptual similarity in the regulation of food and medical products. As the 2012 IOM report *Ensuring Safe Foods and Medical Products Through Stronger Regulatory Systems Abroad* set it out, there are certain attributes that underpin most good regulatory systems (see Box 2-4). The use of science as a basis for policy and the importance of risk as the grounding for regulatory action are central to a good regulatory system (IOM, 2012).

Risk as the Basis for Decisions

Strengthening regulatory systems for both foods and medicines requires a common approach to the scope of work involved. A common framework allows industry, consumers, and other stakeholders to understand where any particular task falls in the regulatory cycle and to see how it relates to other elements of the system. The cornerstone of the regulatory framework, risk can be a difficult concept to convey; it refers to known or suspected threats to health associated with different causes or agents, and risk assessment is the scientific evaluation of such threats (WHO, n.d.-e). For

BOX 2-4
Attributes of Effective Regulatory Systems

- Responsive: Includes the ability to respond in a crisis and to respond to new information and make policy changes when necessary. This characteristic also relates to the agency's ability to stay abreast of current science.
- Outcome-Oriented: Describes the emphasis on product safety outcomes, avoiding prescriptions that would interfere with innovation.
- Predictable: Refers to clarity and openness regarding laws and fairness in their enforcement. Predictability allows for a level playing field among firms in regulated industry.
- Proportional: Allocates controls based on the threat to public health, making sure that products with similar risks are regulated in similar ways. Proportionality depends on risk assessment.
- Independent: Acknowledges that regulatory policy is the result of both scientific and societal forces, but consumer trust and industry's ability to function depend on the agency's ability to operate without political interference.

SOURCE: IOM, 2012.

regulatory agencies the continuous and iterative assessment of the various risks facing a market is essential.

Reducing risks to health in the most cost-effective and efficient way possible is always the goal of regulatory action as resources are scarce and threats are many (IOM and NRC, 2010). While acknowledging that sometimes unforeseen crises arise, in general, risk assessment is a planned part of the agency's strategy, depending mostly on data and risk analysis (IOM and NRC, 2010). Though expert opinion may be necessary, ideally, risk ranking is the result of numeric weighting in analytical modeling (IOM and NRC, 2010). This is not to say that other considerations do not enter into the process: Risks are considered in light of the whole system, including the cost and feasibility of different responses, as well as factors such as market impacts, public perception, and cost (IOM and NRC, 2010).

Openness and communication with a range of stakeholders are cornerstones of a risk-based system; this includes openness about the uncertainty and variability in the data that support regulations, and the other considerations taken into account when making decisions (IOM and NRC, 2010). Finally, any actions taken and decisions made are eventually evaluated, with the results of the evaluation feeding into the iterative process of choosing priorities and acting on them (IOM and NRC, 2010).

Choosing priorities from among the various risks facing an agency is a complicated process because it balances the likelihood and severity of different types of threats (Kowalcyk, 2019). Box 2-5 sets out the steps of a risk-based process. This framework could aid the discussion among regulators in setting priorities for food and medicine safety. Going through the process of identifying and ranking risks, and assessing ways to mitigate them, will help agencies to understand which interventions can be taken at the country level and which ones are candidates for international collaborative action. Cost-benefit and cost-effectiveness analyses can clarify the most effective strategies. Relying on the U.S. Food and Drug Administration's (FDA's) technical decisions on new chemical entities, for example, allows many agencies to use their drug regulatory staff and budget for urgent local needs, like inspection.

Donor programs also need to acknowledge the process of risk ranking in their projects. It can be tempting as a donor to offer solutions to product safety problems without first evaluating the risks in country and considering the range of possible interventions, their cost, and their suitability to the context. Donors could help promote the risk basis in regulatory action by going through a scientific analysis of risk with their counterparts, and designing their interventions accordingly.

Important Groups and Processes

The process of identifying risks and choosing priorities and interventions to counteract them is an iterative process. The process depends, as Box 2-5 makes clear, on data and public consultation. Understanding the nature of such consultation requires an understanding of the main stakeholders regulatory agencies interact with. Figure 2-1 shows relationships among various organizations. Frequent, inclusive interaction with a range of involved parties helps ensure that the regulatory agencies' priorities reflect the will of society, and that their rules are reasonable and serve the goal of improving access to safe and effective medicines and wholesome foods.

Some parties shown in Figure 2-1 have their own convening power, but more often the onus is on the agency to be open and inclusive with its working groups, scientific meetings, information sessions, and other forums (EFSA, n.d.-b). Such consultation is worth the effort. Over time, the agency's priorities change, and changing priorities have implications, especially for industry. Regulatory changes may be better accepted when everyone understands the agency's process and the reasons for its actions. Openness also fosters a respect for the agency's work. The public cannot value the services regulators provide if they are not aware of them.

Figure 2-1 shows how different parties within a system interact. At the same time, food and medicines are global enterprises, and some important dimensions of the process happen at the global level. One process of particular importance for regulators in low- and middle-income countries is the WHO prequalification of medicines.

WHO Prequalification

Prequalification refers to the assessment, inspection, ongoing re-inspection, and quality control WHO provides for certain essential medical products (WHO, 2013). Vaccine prequalification started in 1987; the medicines program started in 2001 as demand for HIV, tuberculosis, and malaria medicines surpassed the production of those manufacturers approved by the FDA and other advanced regulatory authorities (Dellepiane and Wood, 2015; WHO, n.d.-b). In order to give UN agencies and other large procurers a choice of good-quality products for HIV, malaria, and tuberculosis, the WHO provides the equivalent of regulatory assessment for finished medicines, as well as active ingredients and diagnostics; it also maintains 50 labs for quality control (WHO, 2019b, n.d.-b).

Because of prequalification, procurement agencies around the world can be confident they are buying quality-assured medicines, vaccines, diagnostics, and other essential medical products; generic manufacturers have the same safety net in place for their purchase of active ingredients. The

BOX 2-5
Steps in a Risk-Based Regulatory Process

Step 1: Strategic Planning

1. Identify public health objectives related to food safety in consultation with stakeholders.
2. Establish a risk management plan (general and specific strategic plans for meeting public health objectives and for considering and choosing policy interventions to achieve those objectives).
3. Establish metrics with which to measure performance in consultation with stakeholders.

Step 2: Public Health Risk Ranking

1. Develop or select tools (models, measures, or other) for public health risk ranking in consultation with stakeholders.
2. Rank risks based on public health outcomes.
3. Report results to stakeholders and solicit feedback.

Step 3: Targeted Information Gathering on Risks and Consideration of Other Factors That May Influence Decision Making

1. Identify and consider additional criteria upon which risk-based decision making will be based (e.g., public acceptance, cost, controllability, environmental effects, market impacts) in consultation with stakeholders.
2. Conduct targeted information gathering. For each high-priority and/or uncertain risk, determine the need for collection of additional information and implement accordingly:
   a. additional data collection (research, surveillance, survey, baseline data), and
   b. risk assessment (qualitative, quantitative, semi-quantitative).
3. Based on that additional information, identify priority risks for which intervention analysis is needed.

program also has a capacity building element. Regulators from around the world work with WHO staff to review dossiers, evaluate data, and inspect manufacturers together (WHO, 2013). The WHO also provides training and other support to manufacturers and staff at quality control labs (WHO, n.d.-a).

As of early 2019, 546 medicines, the vast majority made in India, have WHO prequalification (WHO, n.d.-c). That designation carries a weight beyond that which licensure from the local regulatory authority would necessarily convey. Although recouping the cost of meeting the international standard can be challenging for some manufacturers, it improves the firms' standing with international buyers (Huang et al., 2018). Food producers may use certification from independent third parties to a similar end.

Step 4: Analysis and Selection of Intervention(s)

1. Identify an appropriate level of protection for each high-priority risk, based on available data and in consultation with stakeholders.
2. Identify intervention options in consultation with stakeholders.
3. Identify the types of technical analysis, including but not limited to risk assessment, needed to evaluate the options; identify performance measures and the initial design of databases.
4. Gather the information necessary to conduct the technical analysis.
5. Choose intervention strategies for implementation using multi-criteria decision analysis.
6. Report results to stakeholders, solicit feedback, and modify intervention strategies if needed.

Step 5: Design of an Intervention Plan

1. Develop a plan for implementing the selected interventions in consultation with stakeholders.
2. Allocate resources and implement interventions.

Step 6: Monitoring and Review

1. Collect and analyze data on evaluation measures selected during strategic planning.
2. Interpret data and evaluate whether the interventions result in the desired intermediate outcomes.
3. Determine whether public health objectives are being met by using performance metrics developed in Step 1 (broad strategic planning).
4. Communicate the results to stakeholders.
5. Review and refine the entire process in an iterative manner as necessary to accomplish both intermediate outcomes and public health objectives so as to achieve continuous improvement over time.

SOURCE: IOM and NRC, 2010.

Third-Party Certification in Food Safety

Food producers may seek certification of their process by an independent, accredited organization as a way to demonstrate their safety standards, or to verify other features of production, such as animal welfare or worker protections, that might command a price premium or market access (Hatanaka et al., 2005). Such an independent organization, being neither part of government nor part of industry, is often called a "third-party" certifier (Lusk et al., 2011). The certification process will usually involve a preassessment application, as well as review of facilities and operations, and a field audit (Hatanaka et al., 2005).

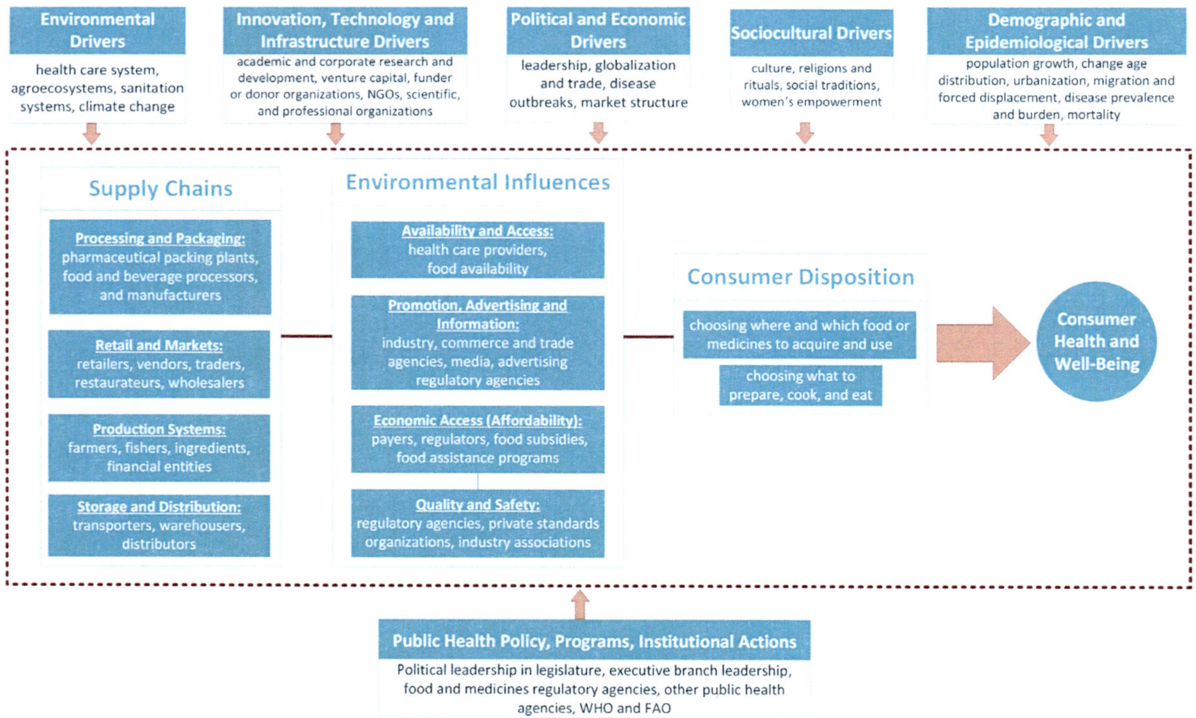

FIGURE 2-1 A conceptual framework of important groups in food and medicines regulation.
NOTE: FAO = Food and Agriculture Organization of the United Nations; NGO = nongovernmental organization; WHO = World Health Organization.
SOURCE: Adapted from HLPE, 2017.

Like WHO prequalification, third-party certification is a consequence of the need for quality assurance when producers work in multiple countries with widely disparate standards and regulatory capacities (Humphrey, 2008). The larger certification programs put considerable emphasis on harmonization of standards and a common approach to audit, making certification something of a de facto regulatory tool in the global food market (Crandall et al., 2012, 2017). Though the standards set by third-party certifiers do not hold the same legal weight as government regulations, the power of the market can compel implementation (Henson and Humphrey, 2010). Supermarket chains, for example, often require third-party certification from their suppliers (Hatanaka et al., 2005; Lee et al., 2012). Furthermore, governments sometimes adapt and reference third-party certifications in their regulations (Henson and Humphrey, 2010).

On one hand, third-party certification allows farmers in countries with limited food regulatory oversight a chance to access lucrative foreign markets, and many do. Over 100,000 operations in 160 countries are certified through the Global Food Safety Initiative alone (GFSI, 2017). Common standards and protocols help minimize the burden of audits and other compliance measures on producers. Compliance with third-party standards can also encourage upgrades to infrastructure and processes with broad benefits to the market (Henson and Humphrey, 2010).

At the same time, meeting the standards, both for the products and for the hygienic process of production, can be prohibitive for small and medium-sized producers in developing countries, for farmers, and for firms operating further downstream, such as exporters (Humphrey, 2008). A recent analysis of the effects of Global GAP certification (one of the most prominent third-party certifications in agriculture) on exports from low- and middle-income countries was mixed (Fiankor et al., 2017). Though certification can be a boon to some parties, there are factors that influence export competitiveness at levels beyond the farm or processing plant (Fiankor et al., 2017). Reliance on third-party standards, especially if those standards are more exacting than laid out in international agreements, can also undermine the authority of the World Trade Organization to adjudicate trade disputes (Henson and Humphrey, 2010).

Furthermore, while attention to standards with an eye to export markets is understandable and necessary for economic growth, it can distort attitudes toward markets meant for domestic consumers. The estimated $410 billion cumulative donor spending on aid for trade between 2006 and 2017 has brought considerable improvements to agriculture, especially in the least developed countries (OECD and WTO, 2019). Almost 40 percent of aid for trade recipients in low- and middle-income countries, and 61 percent of recipients in the least developed countries, identified agriculture as the sector that has seen the most improvement since 2006 (OECD and

WTO, 2019). Despite such success, there are few if any examples of how to improve the safety of food meant for the domestic market (Grace, 2015). As an evaluation in Kenya explained, investments in aquaculture meant a considerable attention directed to fish for the European market, but that "little effort goes to setting and enforcing domestic-market standards" (Abila, 2003).

International Cooperation

A call to strengthen national regulatory agencies is not contrary to the goal of better international cooperation. International cooperation is an essential part of managing the regulatory workload, especially in small or less developed countries. WHO assessments discussed in the next chapter indicated that about three-quarters of WHO member states lack a functional medicines regulatory system (Khadem, 2018). There are no comparable, holistic estimates of the strength of national food control systems, though assessments of different pieces of the system indicate a similar problem. Only about a quarter of low- and middle-income countries have adequately funded veterinary services, for example (Jaffee et al., 2019). Given the regulatory challenges facing every country, cooperation should improve the strength of the national systems.

Even at a cursory level, the diversity and number of stakeholders in food and medicines systems and the global nature of their work make it necessary to cooperate internationally. Agreement on technical guidelines, requirements for registration, and the approach to inspection help lower the burden of regulatory compliance on industry, which in turn can speed market entry and improve access to quality products. These steps also control the burden on the regulatory agency, reducing repetitive work and making more efficient use of staff time. Such efficiency becomes more important when resources are scarce, and most regulatory agencies have considerable strain on their resources (Distrutti and Ramírez, 2018). Even the FDA, perhaps the best supported regulatory agency in the world, has been described as "chronically under-funded" (IOM, 2007). This is why the ability to participate in regional networks and collaborate with other regulators has been cited as one of the minimum functions of a regulatory authority (Rägo and Santoso, 2008).

Some of the best-known examples of regional regulatory cooperation come from Europe. The European Medicines Agency (EMA) is a regional agency for the European Union and the European Economic Area; the European Food Safety Authority serves a similar role for food (EFSA, n.d.-a; EMA, 2016b). The EMA works with a network of regulatory authorities on market surveillance, clinical trials, supervision of manufacturers, and market authorization. Under this system, companies seeking market authorization in Europe can apply for a central authorization for all national markets, multiple authorizations in different countries at the same time, or authorization in one country, with the option to apply for recognition in other European countries (EMA, 2016b). Proposals for similar agencies in Latin America and in Africa are promising but face financial and legal barriers, as well as problems with uneven capacity for enforcement or meeting standards (Distrutti and Ramírez, 2018; Ndomondo-Sigonda et al., 2017). Box 2-6 discusses the proposed African Medicines Agency.

BOX 2-6
African Medicines Agency

In 2018, the African Union unanimously voted to adopt a treaty to establish an African Medicines Agency. The agency will help strengthen regulatory systems and provide access to safer, affordable medicines across the continent. As of August 1, 2019, Algeria, Madagascar, Rwanda, and Sahrawi had officially signed on to the treaty, but it will only come into effect once ratified by 15 member states.

Africa currently has 54 national medicines regulatory authorities but, with varied capacity and limited resources, not all are on the same level of expertise. Each regulatory authority has its own policies, standards, and guidelines. The different regulatory authorities did not work together until the World Bank, the New Partnership for Africa's Development, and the World Health Organization introduced the African Medicines Regulatory Harmonization initiative in 2009, leading to regional efforts to harmonize medicines regulation. For example, the East African Community Medicines Regulatory Harmonization is a regional initiative, where five countries share the cost of regulatory functions by working together to develop registration procedures compatible with internationally recognized standards, and to cooperate on technical matters. The African Medicines Regulatory Harmonization initiative's activities will transition to the African Medicines Agency eventually.

Regional harmonization has already lowered drug prices and approval times. Further improvements are likely as countries avoid redundant testing. Speeding registration, in turn, makes markets more competitive, thereby leading to lower prices and better access. Experts also hope the agency will work with the African Union to help countries build local manufacturing, reducing dependency on imports. Africa's pharmaceutical industry is growing slowly. Currently, there are about 375 medicines manufacturers; they produce only about 10 to 30 percent of the continent's drugs. However, estimates show Africa's pharmaceutical industry increased its value from $4.7 billion in 2003 to $20.8 billion in 2013 and will more than double by 2020.

SOURCES: African Union, 2019a,b; Ndomondo-Sigonda et al., 2017, 2018; NEPAD, 2019; Thomas, 2019; WHO, 2014; Zarocostas, 2018.

At the same time, there are many useful venues for regulatory harmonization and cooperation separate from a formal agency. Industry has initiated some of these networks; others are the product of trade or bilateral relationships. In an effort to understand the extent of bilateral, regional, and global collaboration programs, the International Coalition of Medicines Regulatory Authorities undertook a mapping exercise in 2014. The project report clarifies that the network mapped in Figure 2-2 fluctuates as some organizations change their scope or membership and as new ones form. It also comments on considerable overlap among a confusing array of programs, complicated by "similar initiatives" having "differently-worded objectives," making it difficult to analyze the programs' effectiveness or identify remaining gaps (EMA, 2016a).

There is no analogous mapping for the food systems, perhaps because there is no comparable international coalition for food regulators. This is not to say that similar collaborations for food safety do not happen. The previous chapter described how national and regional food safety labs work together for foodborne disease surveillance through PulseNet, for example. If anything, the collaborations for food safety are more complicated and fractured as they often involve multiple ministries in a single country (e.g., ministries of agriculture, health, and trade). There is also a veterinary component, since food safety includes the health of food-producing animals. Table 2-2 shows examples of some important global and regional food safety organizations and their mandates.

The WHO and the FAO are clear leaders in matters of global health and food safety. The two organizations jointly convene the Codex Alimentarius Commission, the international food standards and guidelines meant to protect health and facilitate trade (FAO, n.d.-a). The agencies also respond to members' requests for food safety support, as in 2000 when concerns raised at the World Health Assembly led the WHO and the FAO to develop the International Food Safety Authorities Network, called INFOSAN (WHO and FAO, 2011). INFOSAN aims to build food safety networks within and among countries thereby improving outbreak response and facilitating recalls when necessary (see Box 2-7). Participating countries (including, at last count, 97 percent of WHO member states) designate at least one contact for emergency response; they also commit to taking part in various food safety activities with other members (Savelli et al., 2019). While these activities may benefit all parties, recent analysis suggests that the countries with good food safety systems to start with are the most active participants (Savelli et al., 2019). The authors, food safety experts from the WHO and a British university, also commented on, "an abundance of regional [food safety] networks and initiatives at various stages of development and utility" and called for a mapping of the networks and the relationships among them (Savelli et al., 2019).

Modern food production is so complex, and supply chains so vast, that even the people with the best knowledge of the system see only pieces of it. The lack of global mapping of food safety stakeholders is itself unfortunate; it is also symptomatic of a larger problem. Food regulators do not have a standing venue to interact with their counterparts in other countries. In this vacuum, it is not clear that any of the multiple regional cooperative ventures or various well-established technical groups are working to maximum efficiency or avoiding redundant effort.

Convening food regulators in regular meetings is also an investment in emergency response. Without a regular opportunity to come together, communication among regulators during a crisis will be at best ad hoc, reinforcing existing relationships. During the 2014 Ebola outbreak in West Africa, for example, the newly formed International Coalition of Medicines Regulatory Authorities committed to cooperation among agencies and with the WHO to speed the review of investigation medicines and vaccines for Ebola (ICMRA, 2014; WHO, 2015). In an international crisis affecting the food supply, valuable response time could be wasted identifying responsible parties in different ministries.

Recommendation 2-1: The Food and Agriculture Organization of the United Nations and the World Health Organization should convene biennial meetings for food safety regulators similar to the International Conference of Drug Regulatory Authorities.

As the UN agencies responsible for global public health and food security, the WHO and the FAO are the best choices to convene the food regulatory meetings suggested. This would be consistent with the agencies' missions to promote health and nutrition and to support governments on matters related to their health and food systems (FAO, n.d.-d; WHO, n.d.-f, n.d.-g). Together the FAO and the WHO convene the Codex Alimentarius Commission and INFOSAN, as well as an expert working group on food additives (FAO, n.d.-a, n.d.-b; WHO, n.d.-d). Convening food regulators is also consistent with previous statements from both organizations on the value of regulatory collaboration (FAO, n.d.-c; ICDRA, 2018; WHO, 2015). The organizations also have existing relationships with ministries that would be asked to designate participants for this activity.

The committee chose the International Conference of Drug Regulatory Authorities (ICDRA) as a model for this recommendation but has no desire to be overly prescriptive in doing so. The WHO first convened ICDRA in 1980 to foster consensus building on drug regulatory questions (FAO, n.d.-c). Now the meetings generally have a few days of programming open to any registered participant, as well as several days of sessions for regulators only (FAO, n.d.-c). ICDRA involves regulators from many levels

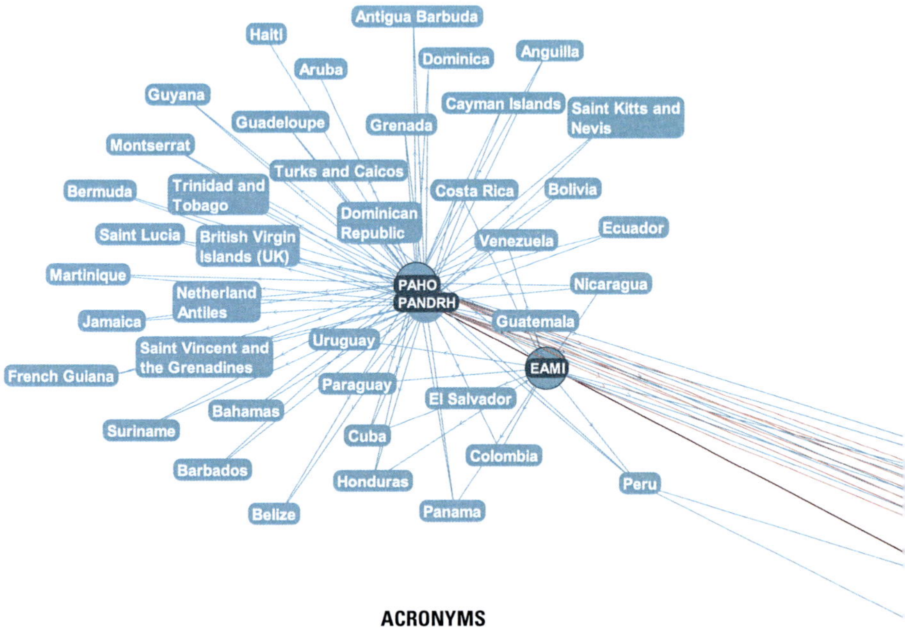

ACRONYMS

AMRH: African Medicines Regulatory Harmonization

APEC: Asia-Pacific Economic Cooperation

ASEAN: Association of Southeast Asian Nations

CEN SAD: Community of Sahel and Saharan States

CIOMS: Council for International Organizations of Medical Sciences

CIRS: The Centre for Innovation in Regulatory Science

DG SANTE: European Commission Health and Food Safety Directorate General

EAC: East African Community

EAMI: Ibero-American Medicines Competent Authorities Network

ECOWAS: Economic Community of West African States

EDQM: European Directorate for the Quality of Medicines

EMA: European Medicines Agency

EMRN: European Medicines Regulatory Network

GCC: Gulf Central Committee for Drug Registration Harmonisation Initiative

ICH: International Council for Harmonisation of Technical Requirements for Pharmaceuticals for Human Use

ICMRA MC: International Coalition of Medicines Regulatory Authorities Management Committee

IGAD: Intergovernmental Authority on Development

IGDRP: International Generic Drug Regulators Pilot

IPRF: International Pharmaceutical Regulators Forum

IRC: International Regulators Consortium Initiative

OCEAC: Organization for the Coordination of the Fight against Endemic Diseases in Central Africa

OECD: Organisation for Economic Co-operation and Development

PAHO: Pan American Health Organization

PANDRH: Pan-American Network for Drug Regulatory Harmonization

PIC/S: Pharmaceutical Inspection Co-operation Scheme

SADC: Southern African Development Community

FIGURE 2-2 Multinational medicines regulatory programs, results of the International Coalition of Medicines Regulatory Authorities' 2014–2015 mapping exercise.
SOURCE: EMA, 2016a.

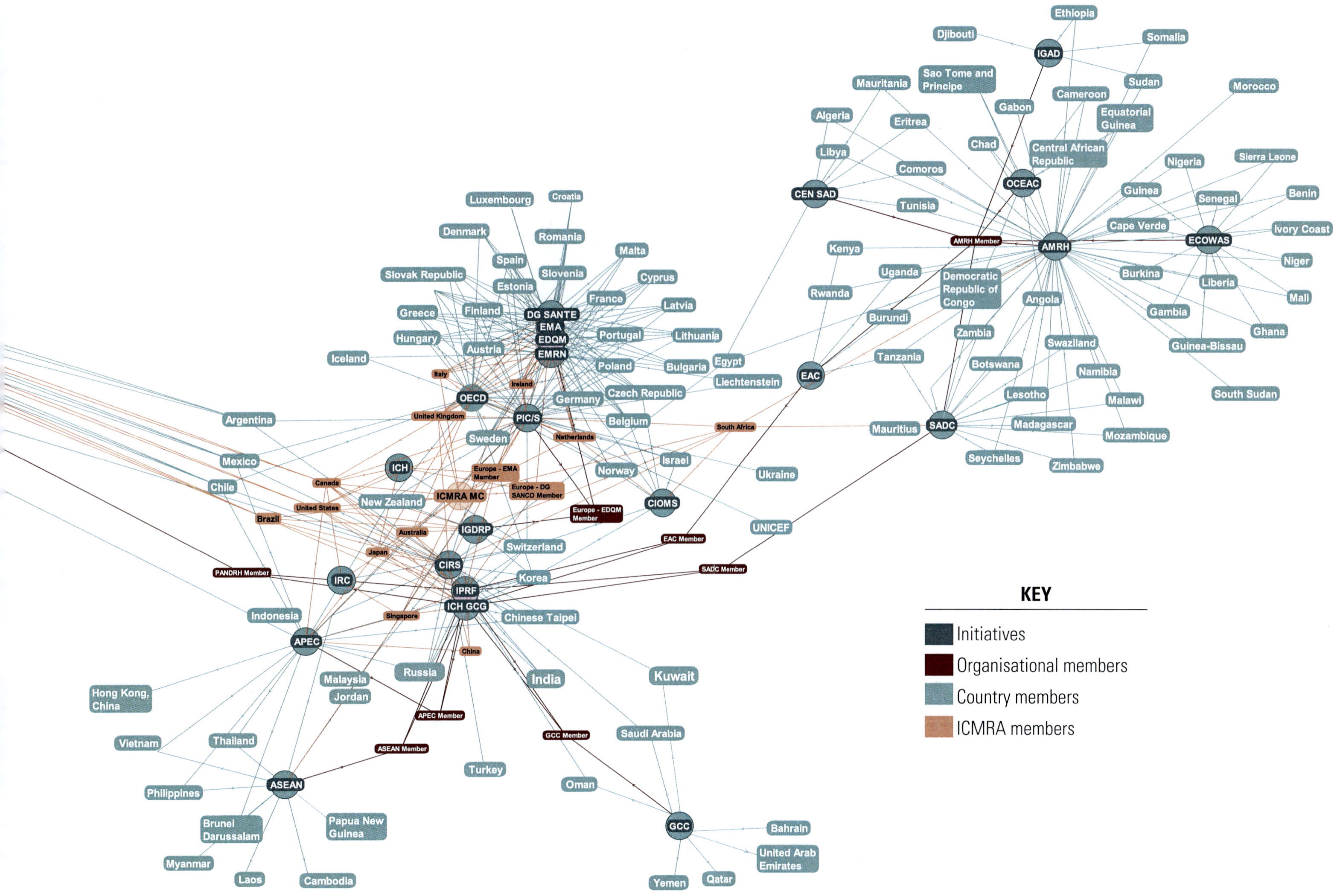
Ethiopia
Djibouti
IGAD
Somalia
Sao Tome and Principe
Mauritania
Sudan
Cameroon
Morocco
Gabon
Equatorial Guinea
Algeria
Eritrea
Chad
Central African Republic
Libya
Comoros
OCEAC
Nigeria
Sierra Leone
CEN SAD
Guinea
Senegal
Benin
Tunisia
Cape Verde
Ivory Coast
AMRH Member
AMRH
ECOWAS
Kenya
Niger
Uganda
Democratic Republic of Congo
Burkina
Liberia
Rwanda
Mali
Angola
Burundi
Gambia
Zambia
Ghana
Swaziland
Guinea-Bissau
Tanzania
Botswana
Namibia
EAC
Lesotho
Malawi
South Sudan
Mauritius
SADC
Madagascar
Mozambique
Seychelles
Zimbabwe
Luxembourg
Croatia
Denmark
Romania
Malta
Spain
Slovak Republic
Slovenia
Cyprus
Estonia
France
Latvia
Greece
Finland
DG SANTE
EMA
EDQM
EMRN
Hungary
Portugal
Lithuania
Austria
Iceland
Poland
Bulgaria
Egypt
Liechtenstein
Italy
Ireland
OECD
Germany
Czech Republic
Argentina
United Kingdom
PIC/S
Belgium
South Africa
Sweden
Netherlands
Mexico
ICH
Israel
Norway
Ukraine
Europe - EMA Member
Canada
Chile
Europe - DG SANCO Member
ICMRA MC
New Zealand
CIOMS
United States
Europe - EDQM Member
Brazil
IGDRP
UNICEF
Australia
Switzerland
Japan
EAC Member
CIRS
SADC Member
PANDRH Member
IRC
Korea
IPRF
ICH GCG
Indonesia
Singapore
Chinese Taipei
APEC
China
Russia
India
Kuwait
Hong Kong, China
Malaysia
Jordan
APEC Member
GCC Member
Saudi Arabia
Vietnam
Thailand
ASEAN Member
Turkey
Oman
Philippines
ASEAN
Brunei Darussalam
Papua New Guinea
GCC
Bahrain
United Arab Emirates
Myanmar
Laos
Cambodia
Yemen
Qatar
KEY
Initiatives
Organisational members
Country members
ICMRA members

of government, technical staff as well as agency leaders. The International Coalition of Medicines Regulatory Authorities, in contrast, involves only heads of agencies and other senior leaders; it is a newer collaboration, and one convened by the leaders themselves (WHO, 2015). Both types of meetings have value. The heads of agencies can best comment on their organizations' strategic direction; they can also direct relatively quick cooperation when necessary. At the same time, there is value to convening technical experts and people at different levels of the agency, who also benefit from the technical discussion and networking (WHO, 2015). For this reason, ICDRA is a good model, and because self-convening may be less realistic for food regulators. There are often multiple government officials of equal rank overseeing food safety, making diffusion of responsibility for convening them more likely.

Regular meetings give various food safety experts the chance to have a predictable and ongoing discussion about current issues. There may be greater political will to support this international discussion now than there has been in the past, driven in part by the estimates of disease burden and cost of foodborne illness discussed in the previous chapter. An inclusive, international discussion on food safety is one way to take advantage of the current interest in the topic.

The increasing scientific and legal complexity of regulatory work and the interconnected nature of the food supply chain make it necessary for food regulators to have a standing, formal venue for technical exchange and cooperation. This forum would be to the benefit of all parties, especially regulators from small countries who may have limited occasions to build relationships with their counterparts abroad.

The programs shown in Table 2-2 and others like them reflect international response to various food safety problems, some existing for a century or more, others only a few years old. These programs and other, sometimes impromptu, collaborations among food regulators have great value, but an inclusive global convening at regular intervals would help ensure they operate to their maximum effectiveness.

Technical experts and scientists today are often criticized for inadequate sharing of information, for working in so-called silos (Lowrey, 2014; Satell, 2017; Talsma, 2016). Some of this perceived narrowness of focus is a consequence of the complexity of their fields and the amount of knowledge generated. In international work, language and distance can magnify the challenge; there are only so many professional connections anyone can be expected to maintain. This is why the convening power of the WHO and the FAO would be a powerful force for collaboration, and one that is needed for food regulators.

TABLE 2-2
A Cross-Section of Multinational Food Safety Programs

	Region or Countries	Role	Website
International Organizations			
Joint FAO and WHO Food Standards Program	Global	Building capacity to prevent, detect, and manage foodborne risks; promoting safe food handling	http://www.fao.org/food-safety/en https://www.who.int/health-topics/food-safety
Inter-American Institute for Cooperation on Agriculture; Agricultural Health, Safety, and Food Quality Program	The Americas	Promoting productive, competitive, and sustainable agriculture through local, regional, and global markets	https://iica.int/en/programs/agricultural-health
Pan America Health Organization Food Safety Regional Program	The Americas	Strengthening national food safety and surveillance systems, risk-based inspection and control systems, and laboratories	https://www.paho.org/hq/index.php?option=com_content&view=article&id=15241:food-safety-is-everyone-s-business&Itemid=1926&lang=en
Caribbean Agricultural Health and Food Safety Agency	Caribbean countries	Supporting national agricultural health and food safety systems in accordance with the Sanitary and Phytosanitary Agreement	https://caricom.org/about-caricom/who-we-are/institutions1/caribbean-agricultural-health-and-food-safety-agency-cahfsa
International Standard Setting Bodies			
Codex Alimentarius Commission	Global	Protecting human health from food safety hazards and facilitating trade	http://www.fao.org/fao-who-codexalimentarius/en
World Animal Health Organization	Global	Improving animal health and facilitating trade	http://www.oie.int
International Plant Protection Convention	Global	Improving plant health and facilitating trade	https://www.ippc.int/en

National Regulatory Units			
European Food Safety Authority	European Union member states	Supporting members' food safety agencies and European Commission institutions with scientific advice and communication on food safety risks	http://www.efsa.europa.eu
Regional Industry Organization			
Food Safety Asia	Various Asia and Middle East	Harmonizing laboratory practices, establishing a regional laboratory network	http://www.foodsafetyasia.net
International Food Safety Capacity Building Organizations or Networks			
World Trade Organization Standard and Trade Development Facility	Global	Improving market access in low- and middle-income countries with attention to sanitary and phytosanitary problems	https://www.standardsfacility.org
Asian Pacific Economic Cooperation; Food Safety Cooperation Forum; Partnership Training Institute Network	APEC countries	Engaging industry and academic food safety experts with regulators for capacity building in food safety	http://fscf-ptin.apec.org
Food Safety Risk Analysis Consortium	Latin America and the Caribbean	Developing and integrating risk analysis in the Americas	https://www.paho.org/panaftosa/index.php?option=com_content&view=article&id=1771:food-safety-risk-analysis-consortium-fsrisk&Itemid=0
JIFSAN	Global	Research to improve food safety and capacity building	https://jifsan.umd.edu

continued

TABLE 2-2 Continued

	Region or Countries	Role	Website
Third-Party Auditors			
Global GAP	Global	Quality and safety standards of good agricultural practices tailored to primary agricultural production	https://www.globalgap.org/uk_en
Global Aquaculture Alliance Seafood	Global	Promote responsible aquaculture practices through education, advocacy, and demonstration	https://www.aquaculturealliance.org
Primus GFS	Global	Auditing of Good Agricultural Practices and Good Manufacturing Practices, as well as Food Safety Management Systems	http://www.primusgfs.com
Monitoring and Data-Sharing Efforts			
Emergency Prevention System for Food Safety	Global	Facilitating rapid sharing of information during food safety emergencies through the International Food Safety Authorities Network	http://www.fao.org/food/food-safety-quality/empres-food-safety/en
International Food Safety Authorities Network (INFOSAN)	Global	Collaborating among food safety authorities for crisis mitigation	https://www.who.int/activities/responding-to-food-safety-emergencies-infosan
PulseNet International	~86 countries worldwide	Public health and food safety laboratory network	http://www.pulsenetinternational.org/international
Research or Trade Associations			
International Association for Food Protection	Individual members from more than 50 countries	Professional association for people working in any aspect of food safety (farming, processing, distribution, etc.)	https://www.foodprotection.org/about

continued

Global Food Safety Initiative	Global	Food industry collaboration to reduce food safety risks and improve efficiency	https://www.mygfsi.com/about-us/about-gfsi/what-is-gfsi.html
Scientific Guidance			
International Commission on Microbiological Specifications of Food	Global	Providing scientific guidance to governments and industry on the microbiological safety of foods	http://www.icmsf.org
HACCP Alliance Capacity Building Activities			
International HACCP Alliance	Meat focused USDA FSIS requirements	Providing a uniform program to assure safer meat and poultry products; hosted by Texas A&M University	http://www.haccpalliance.org/sub/index.html
Seafood HACCP Alliance*	Global	Training program involving representation from FDA, USDA, U.S. Department of Commerce	http://www.afdo.org/page-1186198
Food Safety Preventive Controls Alliance*	U.S. requirement for market access with global implications	Assisting companies producing human and animal food in complying with the U.S. preventive control regulations	https://www.ifsh.iit.edu/fspca
Produce Safety Alliance*	U.S. requirement for market access with global implications	Training and outreach to assist producers and companies with produce safety, public–private partnership hosted by Cornell University	https://producesafetyalliance.cornell.edu/food-safety-modernization-act/produce-safety-rule
Produce Safety Rule-Produce International Partnership*	U.S. requirement for market access with global implications	Building capacity for the produce safety rule internationally	https://jifsan.umd.edu/training/international/courses/pip/description

continued

TABLE 2-2 Continued

	Region or Countries	Role	Website
Sprout Safety Alliance*	U.S. requirement for market access with global implications	Training sprouts producers to enhance understanding and implementation of best practices for improving sprouts safety	https://www.ifsh.iit.edu/ssa
Private Sector Initiatives			
SSAFE	Food companies	Promoting public–private partnerships for food safety and standards	http://www.ssafe-food.org/about-ssafe
Food Industry Asia	Food companies in Asia	Enhancing the industry's role as a partner in the development of scientific food policy in the region	https://foodindustry.asia/home
Regional Networks (including Public and Private Sector)			
African Food Safety Network	Africa Union member states	Collaborating among food safety stakeholders in Africa for public health and trade	https://www.africanfoodsafetynetwork.org
ASEAN Food Safety Network	Southeast Asia	Exchanging information among ASEAN member states	https://www.aseanfoodsafetynetwork.net

* Affiliated with Association of Food and Drug Officials.

BOX 2-7
***Listeria* Outbreak in South Africa**

In July 2017 South African authorities identified an uptick in *listeria* cases; the minister of health officially declared an outbreak in December 2017. Before the outbreak ended in the southern hemisphere winter of 2018, 1,060 people were sickened in what become one of the world's largest documented *listeria* outbreaks. Of the 216 known deaths, at least 80 were infants.

The small public health laboratory responsible for the genome sequencing necessary for tracing the outbreak was new to real-time, whole-genome sequencing in 2017. The volume of samples coming in quickly exceeded staff capacity. With support from the International Food Safety Authorities Network and the Global Outbreak Alert and Response Network, both WHO programs, scientists eventually traced the source of the outbreak to a ready-to-eat processed meat from a factory that produced exports for 15 countries. In March of 2018 the factory was closed and a massive recall began. The ensuing investigation identified weaknesses in the national food safety system at the source factory and at other sites.

Response to the *listeria* outbreak, including at its peak the destruction of about 80 tons of food a day, cost over $800,000. Since then, the WHO and other partners have worked with the South African government to improve foodborne disease surveillance, update food safety laws and regulations, and modernize compliance measures, such as inspections. *Listeria* has also been added to a list of mandatory notifiable diseases in South Africa.

SOURCES: Allam et al., 2018; Murano, 2018; National Institute for Communicable Diseases, 2018; Salama et al., 2018; Whitworth, 2018; WHO, n.d.-h.

REFERENCES

Abila, R. O. 2003. Food safety in food security and food trade—case study: Kenyan fish exports. *2020 Vision* Focus 10.

African Union. 2019a. *List of countries which have signed, ratified/acceded to the treaty for the establishment of the African Medicines Agency*. https://au.int/sites/default/files/treaties/36892-sl-TREATY%20FOR%20THE%20ESTABLISHMENT%20OF%20THE%20AFRICAN%20MEDICINES%20AGENCY.pdf (accessed August 5, 2019).

African Union. 2019b. *The republic of Madagascar signed the treaty for the establishment of the African Medicine Agency (AMA)*, edited by M. Agama-Anyetei. Addis Ababa, Ethiopia: African Union.

Afshin, A., P. J. Sur, K. A. Fay, L. Cornaby, G. Ferrara, J. S. Salama, E. C. Mullany, K. H. Abate, C. Abbafati, Z. Abebe, M. Afarideh, et al. 2019. Health effects of dietary risks in 195 countries, 1990–2017: A systematic analysis for the global burden of disease study 2017. *The Lancet* 393(10184):1958–1972.

Allam, M., N. Tau, S. L. Smouse, P. S. Mtshali, F. Mnyameni, Z. T. H. Khumalo, A. Ismail, N. Govender, J. Thomas, and A. M. Smith. 2018. Whole-genome sequences of *Listeria monocytogenes* sequence type 6 isolates associated with a large foodborne outbreak in South Africa, 2017 to 2018. *Genome Announcement* 6(25).

Baird, J. K. 2013. Malaria caused by *Plasmodium vivax*: Recurrent, difficult to treat, disabling, and threatening to life—the infectious bite preempts these hazards. *Pathogens and Global Health* 107(8):475–479.

Chan, M. 2015. *Universal health coverage: A pro-poor pillar of sustainable development*. Paper presented at International Conference on Universal Health Coverage in the New Development Era, Tokyo, Japan.

Chan, M. 2017. The power of vaccines: Still not fully utilized. In *Ten years in public health, 2007–2017*. Geneva, Switzerland: WHO.

Chan, M., and G. H. Brundtland. 2016. *Universal health coverage: An affordable goal for all*. https://www.who.int/mediacentre/commentaries/2016/universal-health-coverage/en (accessed May 15, 2019).

Chapman, N., A. Doubell, L. Oversteegen, P. Barnsley, V. Chowdhary, G. Rugarabamu, M. Ong, and J. Borri. 2018. Neglected disease research and development: Reaching new heights. *G-FINDER Report*.

Cibulskis, R. E., P. Alonso, J. Aponte, M. Aregawi, A. Barrette, L. Bergeron, C. A. Fergus, T. Knox, M. Lynch, E. Patouillard, S. Schwarte, S. Stewart, and R. Williams. 2016. Malaria: Global progress 2000–2015 and future challenges. *Infectious Diseases of Poverty* 5(1):61.

Cohen, M. J. 2015. U.S. aid to agriculture: Shifting focus from production to sustainable food security. *Penn State Journal of Law & International Affairs* 3(2).

Crandall, P., E. J. Van Loo, C. A. O'Bryan, A. Mauromoustakos, F. Yiannas, N. Dyenson, and I. Berdnik. 2012. Companies' opinions and acceptance of global food safety initiative benchmarks after implementation. *Journal of Food Protection* 75(9):1660–1672.

Crandall, P. G., A. Mauromoustakos, C. A. O'Bryan, K. C. Thompson, F. Yiannas, K. Bridges, and C. Francois. 2017. Impact of the global food safety initiative on food safety worldwide: Statistical analysis of a survey of international food processors. *Journal of Food Protection* 80(10):1613–1622.

Dellepiane, N., and D. Wood. 2015. Twenty-five years of the WHO vaccines prequalification programme (1987–2012): Lessons learned and future perspectives. *Vaccine* 33(1):52–61.

Dieleman, J., C. J. L. Murray, K. C. Margot, M. Campbell, A. Chapin, E. Eldrenkamp, T. Matyasz, A. Micah, A. Reynolds, N. Sadat, M. Schneider, and R. Sorensen. 2016a. Methods annex. In *Financing global health 2016: Development assistance, public and private health spending for the pursuit of universal health coverage*, edited by IHME. Seattle, WA.

Dieleman, J. L., M. T. Schneider, A. Haakenstad, L. Singh, N. Sadat, M. Birger, A. Reynolds, T. Templin, H. Hamavid, A. Chapin, and C. J. Murray. 2016b. Development assistance for health: Past trends, associations, and the future of international financial flows for health. *The Lancet* 387(10037):2536–2544.

Distrutti, M., and I. Ramírez. 2018. Would a regional regulatory agency for health technologies be feasible? In *Gente Saludable*. IDP.

Dunning, C. 2016. 230 indicators approved for SDG agenda. In *Center for Global Development*. https://www.cgdev.org/blog/230-indicators-approved-sdg-agenda (accessed December 7, 2019).

EFSA (European Food Safety Authority). n.d.-a. *How we work*. https://www.efsa.europa.eu/en/about/howwework (accessed October 4, 2019).

EFSA. n.d.-b. *Stakeholder engagement*. http://www.efsa.europa.eu/en/partnersnetworks/stakeholder (accessed July 16, 2019).

EMA (European Medicines Agency). 2016a. *Connecting the dots towards global knowledge of the international medicine regulatory landscape: Mapping of international initiatives*. https://www.ema.europa.eu/en/documents/leaflet/connecting-dots-towards-global-knowledge-international-medicine-regulatory-landscape-mapping_en.pdf (accessed September 5, 2019).

EMA. 2016b. *The European regulatory system for medicines: A consistent approach to medicines regulation across the European Union*. London, UK: European Medicines Agency. https://www.ema.europa.eu/en/documents/leaflet/european-regulatory-system-medicines-european-medicines-agency-consistent-approach-medicines_en.pdf (accessed September 11, 2019).

Eze, S., W. Ijomah, and T. C. Wong. 2019. Accessing medical equipment in developing countries through remanufacturing. *Journal of Remanufacturing* 9(3):207–233.

Fagotto, E. 2013. Private roles in food safety provision: The law and economics of private food safety. *European Journal of Law and Economics* 32.

FAO (Food and Agriculture Organization of the United Nations). 2003. *Elements of a national food control system*. http://www.fao.org/3/y8705e/y8705e04.htm (accessed May 24, 2019).

FAO. n.d.-a. *About Codex Alimentarius*. http://www.fao.org/fao-who-codexalimentarius/about-codex/en (accessed July 16, 2019).

FAO. n.d.-b. *Chemical risks and JECFA*. http://www.fao.org/food/food-safety-quality/scientific-advice/jecfa/en (accessed July 15, 2019).

FAO. n.d.-c. *Collaboration between countries*. http://www.fao.org/ag/againfo/programmes/en/empres/gemp/empres/emp3/3510-countries.html (accessed July 16, 2019).

FAO. n.d.-d. *What we do*. http://www.fao.org/about/what-we-do/en (accessed July 15, 2019).

Fiankor, D., I. Flachsbarth, A. Masood, and B. Brummer. 2017. *Does GlobalGAP certification promote agricultural exports?* Paper presented at 19th Annual European Study Group Conference, July 27, Florence, Italy.

Frenk, J., and D. de Ferranti. 2012. Universal health coverage: Good health, good economics. *The Lancet* 380(9845):862–864.

Frenk, J., O. Gomez-Dantes, and S. Moon. 2014. From sovereignty to solidarity: A renewed concept of global health for an era of complex interdependence. *The Lancet* 383(9911):94–97.

GFSI (Global Food Safety Initiative). 2017. *GFSI on strategic partnerships to enhance the safety of imported foods*. https://mygfsi.com/2017/02/21/gfsi-on-strategic-partnerships-to-enhance-the-safety-of-imported-fods (accessed February 13, 2020).

GFSP (Global Food Safety Partnership). 2019. *Food safety in Africa: Past endeavors and future directions.* Washington, DC: World Bank Group.

Global Burden of Disease Pediatrics Collaboration. 2016. Global and national burden of diseases and injuries among children and adolescents between 1990 and 2013: Findings from the global burden of disease 2013 study. *JAMA Pediatrics* 170(3):267–287.

Grace, D. 2015. Food safety in low and middle income countries. *International Journal of Environmental Research and Public Health* 12(9):10490–10507.

Hatanaka, M., C. Bain, and L. Busch. 2005. Third-party certification in the global agrifood system. *Food Policy* 30(3):354–369.

Henson, S., and J. Humphrey. 2010. Understanding the complexities of private standards in global agri-food chains as they impact developing countries. *The Journal of Development Studies* 46(9):1628–1646.

HLPE (High Level Panel of Experts on Food Security and Nutrition of the Food and Agriculture Organization of the United Nations). 2017. *Nutrition and food systems: A report by high level panel of experts on food security and nutrition of the committee on world food security.* Rome, Italy: FAO.

Hogan, D. R., G. A. Stevens, A. R. Hosseinpoor, and T. Boerma. 2018. Monitoring universal health coverage within the sustainable development goals: Development and baseline data for an index of essential health services. *The Lancet Global Health* 6(2):e152–e168.

Huang, Y., K. Pan, D. Peng, and A. Stergachis. 2018. A qualitative assessment of the challenges of WHO prequalification for anti-malarial drugs in China. *Malaria Journal* 17(1):149.

Hug, L., M. Alexander, D. You, and L. Alkema. 2019. National, regional, and global levels and trends in neonatal mortality between 1990 and 2017, with scenario-based projections to 2030: A systematic analysis. *The Lancet Global Health* 7(6):e710–e720.

Humphrey, J. 2008. *Private standards, small farmers and donor policy: EUREPGAP in Kenya,.* London, UK: Institute of Development Studies.

ICDRA (International Conference of Drug Regulatory Authorities). 2018. *Smart safety surveillance: A life-cycle approach to promoting safety of medical products.* Paper read at 18th International Conference of Drug Regulatory Authorities, Dublin, Ireland.

ICMRA (International Coalition of Medicines Regulatory Authorities). 2014. *Consolidated joint ICMRA statement Ebola.* http://www.icmra.info/docs/Consolidated_Joint_ICMRA_statement_Ebola.pdf (accessed February 19, 2020).

Institute for Health Metrics and Evaluation. 2017. *Findings from the global burden of disease study 2017.* Seattle, WA: IHME.

IOM (Institute of Medicine). 2007. *Challenges for the FDA: The future of drug safety: Workshop summary.* Washington, DC: The National Academies Press.

IOM. 2012. *Ensuring safe foods and medical products through stronger regulatory systems abroad.* Washington, DC: The National Academies Press.

IOM. 2014. *Investing in global health systems: Sustaining gains, transforming lives.* Washington, DC: The National Academies Press.

IOM and NRC (National Research Council). 2010. *Enhancing food safety: The role of the Food and Drug Administration.* Washington, DC: The National Academies Press.

Jaffee, S., S. Henson, L. Unnevehr, D. Grace, and E. Cassou. 2019. *The safe food imperative : Accelerating progress in low- and middle-income countries. Agriculture and food series.* Washington, DC: World Bank.

Khadem, A. 2018. *Building regulatory capacity in countries to improve the regulation of health products.* https://www.who.int/medicines/technical_briefing/tbs/TBS2018_RSS_Capacity_Building_CRSgroup.pdf?ua=1 (accessed February 13, 2020).

Kharas, H. 2017. *The unprecedented expansion of the global middle class: An update.* Washington, DC: The Brookings Institution.

Kowalcyk, B. 2019. *Developing a risk-based framework for food safety decision-making in low and middle income countries*. Paper presented at Stronger Food and Drug Regulatory Systems Abroad, April 3, Washington, DC.

Lagomarsino, G., A. Garabrant, A. Adyas, R. Muga, and N. Otoo. 2012. Moving towards universal health coverage: Health insurance reforms in nine developing countries in africa and asia. *The Lancet* 380(9845):933–943.

Lee, J., G. Gereffi, and J. Beauvais. 2012. Global value chains and agrifood standards: Challenges and possibilities for smallholders in developing countries. *Proceedings of the National Academy of Sciences of the United States of America* 109(31):12326–12331.

Lowrey, A. 2014. World Bank revamping is rattling employees. *The New York Times*, May 27, 2014. https://www.nytimes.com/2014/05/28/business/international/world-bank-revamping-is-rattling-employees.html?login=smartlock&auth=login-smartlock (accessed February 13, 2020).

Lusk, J. L., J. Roosen, J. F. Shogren, J. A. Caswell, and S. M. Anders. 2011. Private versus third party versus government labeling. In *The Oxford handbook of the economics of food consumption and policy*. New York: Oxford University Press.

Moon, S., and O. Omole. 2017. Development assistance for health: Critiques, proposals and prospects for change. *Health Economics, Policy, and Law* 12(2):207–221.

Moon, S., J. A. Rottingen, and J. Frenk. 2017. Global public goods for health: Weaknesses and opportunities in the global health system. *Health Economics, Policy, and Law* 12(2):195–205.

Moreno-Serra, R., and P. C. Smith. 2012. Does progress towards universal health coverage improve population health? *The Lancet* 380(9845):917–923.

Murano, E. 2018. *Listeria* in South Africa: Lessons learned. In *Food Safety Net Services*. http://fsns.com/news/listeria-in-south-africa (accessed December 7, 2019)

Murray, C. J., K. F. Ortblad, C. Guinovart, S. S. Lim, T. M. Wolock, D. A. Roberts, E. A. Dansereau, N. Graetz, R. M. Barber, J. C. Brown, H. Wang, H. C. Duber, et al. 2014. Global, regional, and national incidence and mortality for HIV, tuberculosis, and malaria during 1990–2013: A systematic analysis for the global burden of disease study 2013. *The Lancet* 384(9947):1005–1070.

Narrod, C., A. Stumpf, and X. Dou. 2019 (unpublished). Harnessing public–private partnerships for data sharing to measure the impact of food safety capacity building.

National Institute for Communicable Diseases. 2018. *Listeriosis update*. http://www.nicd.ac.za/listeriosis_update (accessed June 26, 2019).

Ndomondo-Sigonda, M., J. Miot, S. Naidoo, A. Dodoo, and E. Kaale. 2017. Medicines regulation in Africa: Current state and opportunities. *Society of Pharmaceutical Medicine* 31(6):383–397.

Ndomondo-Sigonda, M., M. Agama-Anyetei, G. Mahlangu, and H. Mkandawire. 2018. African Medicines Agency Establishment Treaty adopted by African ministers of health. *Global Forum* 10(7).

NEPAD (New Partnership for Africa's Development). 2019. *AUDA-NEPAD and WHO, joint secretariat of the African Medicines Regulatory Harmonisation initiative*. http://www.nepad.org/news/auda-nepad-and-who-joint-secretariat-african-medicines-regulatory-harmonisation (accessed July 15, 2019).

ODI (Overseas Development Institute). 2012. *Measuring aid to agriculture and food security*. https://www.odi.org/publications/6328-aid-agriculture-food-security-measurement (accessed December 7, 2019).

OECD (Organisation for Economic Co-operation and Development). n.d. *Regulatory reform and innovation*. https://www.oecd.org/sti/inno/2102514.pdf (accessed November 18, 2019).

OECD and WTO (World Trade Organization). 2019. *Aid for trade facts and figures*. https://www.wto.org/english/res_e/booksp_e/aid4trade19_facts_e.pdf (accessed September 30, 2019).

Ottersen, T., S. Moon, and J. A. Rottingen. 2017. The challenge of middle-income countries to development assistance for health: Recipients, funders, both or neither? *Health Economics, Policy, and Law* 12(2):265–284.

PAHO (Pan American Health Organization). 2002. *Public health in the Americas: Conceptual renewal, performance assessment, and bases for action*. Washington, DC: PAHO.

PAHO and WHO (World Health Organization). 2016. *Region of the Americas is declared free of measles*. https://www.paho.org/hq/index.php?option=com_content&view=article&id=12528:region-americas-declared-free-measles&Itemid=1926&lang=en (accessed November 25, 2019).

Rägo, L., and B. Santoso. 2008. Drug regulation: History, present and future. In *Drug benefits and risks: International textbook of clinical pharmacology, revised 2nd edition*, edited by C. J. van Boxtel, B. Santoso, and I. R. Edwards. Amsterdam, Netherlands: IOS Press.

Sachs, J. D. 2012. Achieving universal health coverage in low-income settings. *The Lancet* 380(9845):944–947.

Salama, P. J., P. K. B. Embarek, J. Bagaria, and I. S. Fall. 2018. Learning from *Listeria*: Safer food for all. *The Lancet* 391(10137):2305–2306.

Satell, G. 2017. *Breaking down silos is a myth, do this instead: Horizontal connections are what's important*. https://www.inc.com/greg-satell/breaking-down-silos-is-a-myth-do-this-instead.html (accessed July 15, 2019).

Savelli, C. J., A. Bradshaw, P. Ben Embarek, and C. Mateus. 2019. The FAO/WHO international food safety authorities network in review, 2004–2018: Learning from the past and looking to the future. *Foodborne Pathogens and Disease* 16(7):480–488.

Schensul, D. 2016. *SDG 3: Target 3.8: Indicator 3.8.1 definitions, metadata, trends, work plan, and challenges*. Paper presented at Regional Meeting: Enhancing capacity for the integration of the ICPD agenda into SDG adaptation and review processes in Eastern Europe and Central Asia, November 2–4, Geneva, Switzerland.

Talsma, T. 2016. *Eliminating silos in regionally distributed organizations to encourage knowledge sharing*. Senior project paper 8. Allendale, MI: Grand Valley State University.

The Economist. 2015. *It's not what you spend; how to make aid to poor countries work better*. https://www.economist.com/international/2015/05/23/its-not-what-you-spend (accessed May 24, 2019).

The Economist. 2016. *Misplaced charity: Aid is best spent in poor, well-governed countries. That isn't where it goes*. https://www.economist.com/international/2016/06/11/misplaced-charity (accessed May 24, 2019).

The Lancet. 2017. Life, death, and disability in 2016. *The Lancet* 390(10100):1083.

Thomas, D. 2019. *African pharma: A prescription for success*. https://africanbusinessmagazine.com/sectors/health-sectors/african-pharma-a-prescription-for-success (accessed June 25, 2019).

Tzioumis, E., M. C. Kay, M. E. Bentley, and L. S. Adair. 2016. Prevalence and trends in the childhood dual burden of malnutrition in low- and middle-income countries, 1990–2012. *Public Health and Nutrition* 19(8):1375–1388.

UHC2030 (Universal Health Coverage). 2018. *SDG indicator 3.8.1: Measure what matters*. https://www.uhc2030.org/news-events/uhc2030-news/sdg-indicator-3-8-1-measure-what-matters-465653 (accessed May 16, 2019).

UHC2030. 2019. *The UN high-level meeting (UN HLM) on universal health coverage, 23 September 2019, New York*. https://www.uhc2030.org/un-hlm-2019 (accessed May 15, 2019).

UN (United Nations). 2012. *67/l.36 Global health and foreign policy*. https://www.un.org/ga/search/view_doc.asp?symbol=A/67/L.36 (accessed May 15, 2019).

UN. 2015. *Millennium development goals*. https://www.un.org/millenniumgoals (accessed May 15, 2019).

UN. 2016. *Final list of proposed sustainable development goal indicators*. https://sustainabledevelopment.un.org/content/documents/11803Official-List-of-Proposed-SDG-Indicators.pdf (accessed May 16, 2019).

UN. 2018a. *International Universal Health Coverage Day 12 December*. https://www.un.org/en/events/universal-health-coverage (accessed May 15, 2019).

UN. 2018b. *Sustainable development goals*. https://sustainabledevelopment.un.org/sdgs (accessed May 15, 2019).

UN. 2019a. *Political declaration of the high-level meeting on universal health coverage "universal health coverage: Moving together to build a healthier world."* https://www.un.org/pga/73/wp-content/uploads/sites/53/2019/05/UHC-Political-Declaration-zero-draft.pdf (accessed May 15, 2019).

UN. 2019b. *SDG indicators: Metadata repository*. https://unstats.un.org/sdgs/metadata (accessed May 16, 2019).

United Nations Inter-agency Group for Child Mortality Estimation. 2018. *Levels & trends in child mortality: Report 2018, estimates developed by the un inter-agency group for child mortality estimation*. New York: United Nations Children's Fund.

Valin, H., R. D. Sands, D. van der Mensbrugghe, G. C. Nelson, H. Ahammad, E. Blanc, B. Bodirsky, S. Fujimori, T. Hasegawa, P. Havlik, E. Heyhoe, P. Kyle, D. Mason-D'Croz, S. Paltsev, S. Rolinski, A. Tabeau, H. van Meijl, M. von Lampe, and D. Willenbockel. 2014. The future of food demand: Understanding differences in global economic models. *Agricultural Economics* 45(1):51–67.

Wagstaff, A., G. Flores, J. Hsu, M. F. Smitz, K. Chepynoga, L. R. Buisman, K. van Wilgenburg, and P. Eozenou. 2018a. Progress on catastrophic health spending in 133 countries: A retrospective observational study. *The Lancet Global Health* 6(2):e169–e179.

Wagstaff, A., G. Flores, M. F. Smitz, J. Hsu, K. Chepynoga, and P. Eozenou. 2018b. Progress on impoverishing health spending in 122 countries: A retrospective observational study. *The Lancet Global Health* 6(2):e180–e192.

Whitworth, J. 2018. *South Africa declares end to largest ever* Listeria *outbreak*. https://www.foodsafetynews.com/2018/09/south-africa-declares-end-to-largest-ever-listeria-outbreak (accessed June 24, 2019).

WHO (World Health Organization). 2003. *Effective medicines regulation: Ensuring safety, efficacy and quality.* Geneva, Switzerland: World Health Organization.

WHO. 2013. *Prequalification of medicines by WHO*. https://www.who.int/news-room/fact-sheets/detail/prequalification-of-medicines-by-who (accessed June 19, 2019).

WHO. 2014. WHO support for medicines regulatory harmonization in africa: Focus on East African community. *WHO Drug Information* 28(1):11–15. Geneva, Switzerland: World Health Organization.

WHO. 2015. Regulatory collaboration, the International Coalition of Medicines Regulatory Authorities (ICMRA). *WHO Drug Information* 29(1):3–6. Geneva, Switzerland: World Health Organization.

WHO. 2017. *Integrating neglected tropical diseases into global health and development: Fourth WHO report on neglected tropical diseases*. Geneva, Switzerland: World Health Organization.

WHO. 2018a. *Essential public health functions, health systems and health security: Developing conceptual clarity and a WHO roadmap for action*. Geneva, Switzerland: World Health Organization.

WHO. 2018b. *Global tuberculosis report 2018*. Geneva, Switzerland: World Health Organization.

WHO. 2019a. *Distribution of R&D funding flows for neglected diseases (g-finder), by source and type of funding*. https://www.who.int/research-observatory/monitoring/inputs/neglected_diseases_source/en (accessed May 28, 2019).

WHO. 2019b. *WHO list of prequalified quality control laboratories: 47th editon*. https://extranet.who.int/prequal/sites/default/files/documents/PQ_QCLabsList_27.pdf (accessed October 2, 2019).

WHO. 2020. *Universal health coverage day*. https://www.who.int/life-course/news/events/uhc-day/en (accessed January 16, 2020).

WHO. n.d.-a. *Capacity building*. https://extranet.who.int/prequal/content/capacity-building-0 (accessed July 16, 2019).

WHO. n.d.-b. *Key facts about the WHO prequalification project*. https://www.who.int/3by5/prequal/en (accessed July 16, 2019).

WHO. n.d.-c. *Medicines/finished pharmaceutical products*. https://extranet.who.int/prequal/content/prequalified-lists/medicines (accessed February 13, 2020).

WHO. n.d.-d. *Responding to food safety emergencies (INFOSAN)*. https://www.who.int/activities/responding-to-food-safety-emergencies-infosan (accessed July 15, 2019).

WHO. n.d.-e. *Risk assessment*. https://www.who.int/foodsafety/micro/riskassessment/en (accessed May 29, 2019).

WHO. n.d.-f. *What we do*. https://www.who.int/about/what-we-do (accessed July 15, 2019).

WHO. n.d.-g. *WHO's work with countries, cooperation with countries*. https://www.who.int/country-cooperation/en (accessed July 15, 2019).

WHO. n.d.-h. *WHO congratulates South Africa on the end of the world's largest listeriosis outbreak*. https://www.afro.who.int/news/who-congratulates-south-africa-end-worlds-largest-listeriosis-outbreak (accessed July 17, 2019).

WHO and FAO (Food and Agriculture Organization of the United Nations). 2011. *The International Food Safety Authorities Network (INFOSAN) progress report 2004–2010*.

WHO and World Bank. 2015. *Tracking universal health coverage: First global monitoring report*. Geneva, Switzerland: World Health Organization.

WHO and World Bank. 2017. *Tracking universal health coverage: 2017 global monitoring report*. Geneva, Switzerland: World Health Organization.

Wirtz, V. J., H. V. Hogerzeil, A. L. Gray, M. Bigdeli, C. P. de Joncheere, M. A. Ewen, M. Gyansa-Lutterodt, S. Jing, V. L. Luiza, R. M. Mbindyo, H. Möller, C. Moucheraud, B. Pécoul, L. Rägo, A. Rashidian, D. Ross-Degnan, P. N. Stephens, Y. Teerawattananon, E. F. M. 't Hoen, A. K. Wagner, P. Yadav, and M. R. Reich. 2017. Essential medicines for universal health coverage. *The Lancet* 389(10067):403–476.

World Bank. 2015. *World Bank forecasts global poverty to fall below 10% for first time; major hurdles remain in goal to end poverty by 2030*. http://www.worldbank.org/en/news/press-release/2015/10/04/world-bank-forecasts-global-poverty-to-fall-below-10-for-first-time-major-hurdles-remain-in-goal-to-end-poverty-by-2030 (accessed May 24, 2019).

World Bank. n.d. *Poverty headcount ratio at $1.90 a day (2011 ppp) (% of population)*. https://data.worldbank.org/indicator/SI.POV.DDAY?locations (accessed May 28, 2019).

Zarocostas, J. 2018. Health ministers adopt African Medicines Agency Treaty. *The Lancet* 391(10137):2310.

3

Global Efforts to Strengthen Regulatory Systems

The recent work of the Food Epidemiology Research Group, the World Bank's *The Safe Food Imperative*, and World Health Organization (WHO) publications on falsified and substandard medicines discussed earlier in this report have had the welcome consequence of drawing attention to regulatory systems problems in low- and middle-income countries. Unsafe food kills over 400,000 people a year, disproportionately children, and costs the world's economy $110 billion in both treatment and lost productivity (Jaffee et al., 2019; WHO, 2015). Falsified and substandard medicines cause about 70,000 excess deaths from childhood pneumonia and account for between 2 and 5 percent of malaria deaths in sub-Saharan Africa alone (WHO, 2017). These are powerful numbers that put the public health significance of unsafe food and poor quality medicines in context. These problems take a toll on developing countries similar to that of HIV, malaria, or tuberculosis.

Better clarity on the size of a global problem should engender a proportionate, global response. Yet, much of the immediate reaction to these reports has emphasized local solutions from the need for African consumers to demand food safety from their governments to the responsibility of national governments for market surveillance and enforcement of regulations (Crossette, 2019; UN, 2017; Whitworth, 2018). No one could deny the importance of the consumer, the regulator, or the political leader in solving this problem, but their actions cannot reach their full value if the global environment does not foster product safety.

Global health and development organizations, including the United Nations (UN) agencies, development banks, and major donors have considerable power to influence policy in ways that encourage functional regulatory systems. This chapter recommends actions these organizations[1] can take to strengthen product safety systems. It also discusses how circumstances beyond the control of a single country influence local markets for food and medical products.

THE ROLE OF AID

As the previous chapter stated, donor assistance for health now makes up a relatively small piece of total health spending in most of the world, making the effectiveness of the remaining contribution crucial, especially to the donors. Since the 1990s, if not earlier, there has been concern that the manner in which foreign aid is delivered can do unintentional harm in recipient countries. Such problems can be logistical, as when donor contributions are redundant or not in line with local needs. Coordinating donations from multiple sources also adds to the burden on scarce accountants and managers in recipient countries.

Aid effectiveness has been a particular interest of the Organisation for Economic Co-operation and Development (OECD), which convened the 2005 forum that produced the Paris Declaration on Aid Effectiveness (OECD, n.d.-a). The Paris Declaration set out a road map for the future of aid, emphasizing coordination among donors, aligning with the host country's priorities, and the need for donors and recipients of aid to hold each other accountable (OECD, n.d.-a). Subsequent initiatives in the same vein (the 2007 International Health Partnership, the 2008 Accra Agenda for Action, the 2011 Busan Partnership for Effective Cooperation) have reaffirmed these principles and the goal of making aid more predictable, efficient, and useful (Osondu and Yamey, 2019).

Untying Aid and Building Institutions

Aid effectiveness has two features especially relevant to the discussion of regulatory systems. The first is the untying of aid, meaning removing conditions that required aid recipients to procure goods and services through the donor country (OECD, n.d.-b). Such conditions can increase the cost of a project 15 to 30 percent, more if food is procured (Meeks, 2017; OECD, n.d.-b). Procurement conditions in development also limit the usefulness of foreign assistance in building the local economy, something especially shortsighted in the case of food and medical products (Meeks, 2017).

Members of the OECD's Development Assistance Committee have committed to untying aid in the least developed countries and in heavily

[1] Described increasingly as "development partners" (Digital Campus Moodle, 2016).

indebted poor countries; progress toward this goal has been consistent and good (OECD, 2019). Despite recent drops, over 87 percent of relevant aid is untied (OECD, 2017). Fully realizing the spirit of the move away from tied procurement, meaning using donor money to build the local economy, will depend on functional regulatory systems to ensure that products produced locally are of good quality (IADB, 2017).

Building regulatory systems is part of a larger question of institution building, mentioned in the Paris Declaration and Accra Agenda (OECD, n.d.-a; UN, n.d.). To better build institutions, donors committed to channeling 55 percent of aid through local financial systems, though this goal has not been met (OECD, 2015).

Despite a theoretical commitment to institution building, donors, especially bilateral donors, continue to spend in ways that, far from supporting institutional development, can undermine it by setting up parallel management and reporting systems for their projects, for example (de Ronzio, 2016). Instead of investing in the long-term development of capacity, something of a fuzzy concept, most aid projects measure outcomes they can realistically expect to change within a few years (de Ronzio, 2016).

Donors, for their part, have understandable reasons for such action. In some ways, ceding control of the taxpayers' money to a foreign government, especially one not known for strong financial management, could be seen as poor stewardship. An interest in measurable, short-term outcomes, things like the number of bednets delivered or farmers trained in Good Agricultural Practices, comes from a culture of accountability (de Ronzio, 2016). Decision makers in donor countries know that they will have to justify their spending to the public, driving a tension between "results today and capacity tomorrow" (Kenny, 2016). As a World Bank analysis explained, "in their need to show results, donors ... shirk on provision of the public sector human and organizational infrastructure essential for the country's overall long-term development" (Knack and Rahman, 2007).

Benchmarking Regulatory Systems

Recent attention to measuring the capacity of regulatory systems could help adjust the donor calculation to encourage spending on building institutions, specifically on building the institutions that protect the safety of food and medicines, thereby increasing options for local procurement. A valid benchmarking tool can put clear parameters on the otherwise amorphous concept of institutional capacity. There is already good consensus on the jobs regulatory authorities need to do to ensure product quality, as reflected in international assessment tools.

The World Health Organization Global Benchmarking Tool for National Medicines Regulatory Systems

The Global Benchmarking Tool was developed in response to a 2014 World Health Assembly resolution on strengthening regulatory systems for medical products (WHA, 2014). The current iteration of the tool was developed over several years after consultation with WHO member states and with the public, as well as meetings with experts from regulatory authorities around the world (WHO, n.d.-g). The tool can be used to evaluate agencies regulating medicines and biologics; expansion to include devices, diagnostics, blood, and blood products are in development (WHO, n.d.-g).

Results of the benchmarking assessment designate medicines and biologics regulatory authorities at one of four maturity levels, a concept carried over from the International Organization for Standardization's (ISO's) guidance on quality of organizations. Figure 3-1 describes these levels, linking them to ISO standards, and noting the level 3 cut point that countries are meant to aim for.

In short, WHO benchmarking identifies the strengths and areas of improvement of regulatory authorities and their overall maturity level. The benchmarking process involves independent assessors' nine key functions: national regulatory systems (generally dealing with legal provisions and enforcement), registration and market authorization, vigilance, market surveillance and control, licensing of establishments, regulatory inspections, laboratory testing, oversight of clinical trials, and lot release of vaccines.[2] During the evaluation, the assessors collect information on 268 indicators of the system's function, all of which are described in detail on the WHO website (Khadem, 2018; WHO, n.d.-g). The agency's relative performance in each area gives its leaders indication of where to focus efforts for improvement. Figure 3-2 gives graphical representation of a hypothetical agency's performance; the red line indicating the level three target, making it easier to visualize the agency's relative gaps.

The outcome of the benchmarking assessment informs a 5-year institutional development plan wherein agencies identify how they can improve on their relative weaknesses (Khadem, 2018; Ward, 2019). This plan should have provisions for annual and semi-annual progress reviews; an assessment team will review progress after about 2.5 years, and after 5 years, the benchmarking exercise will be repeated (Khadem, 2018).

[2] The first eight functions are common to all medical products regulation, but lot release, which applies only to vaccines, is sometimes described as the "non-common" function.

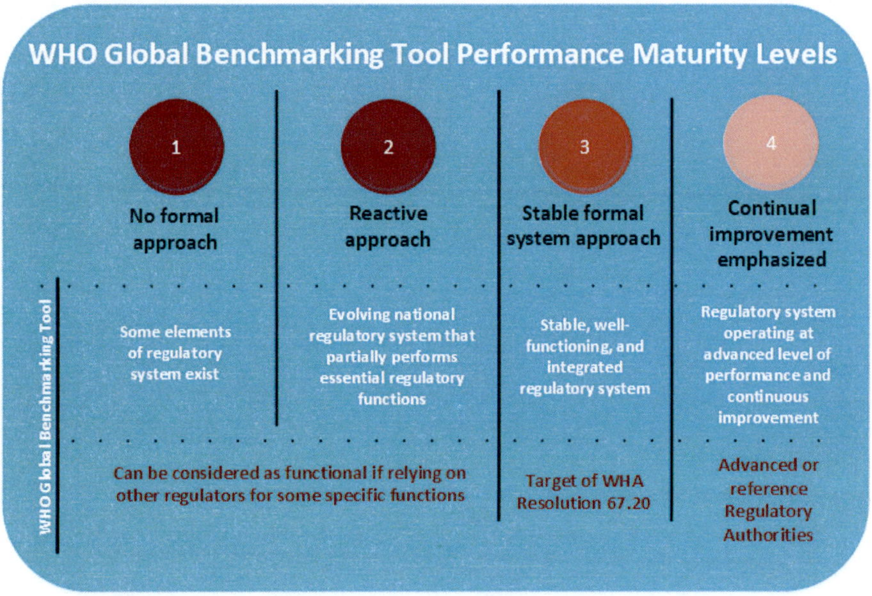

FIGURE 3-1 WHO Global Benchmarking Tool performance levels.
NOTE: ISO = International Organization for Standardization; WHA = World Health Assembly; WHO = World Health Organization.
SOURCE: Khadem, 2018.

Food Safety Systems Benchmarking

Assessment of the food safety system is more complicated than the analogous process for medicines, especially in low- and middle-income countries where there may be multiple systems serving different markets. One system is that of the informal market, over which regulators have, almost by definition, no control. (Informal markets are discussed further in Chapter 5.) Many low- and middle-income countries also have a thriving production system for food exports. Between 2001 and 2016, export of high-value foods (animal-source foods, fresh produce, spices, and nuts) from low- and middle-income countries increased four-fold (Jaffee et al., 2019). This thriving market is credited to improvements in production and efficiency, as well as in the management of the export food market, with both the government and the private sector investing in meeting requirements for market access (Jaffee et al., 2019).

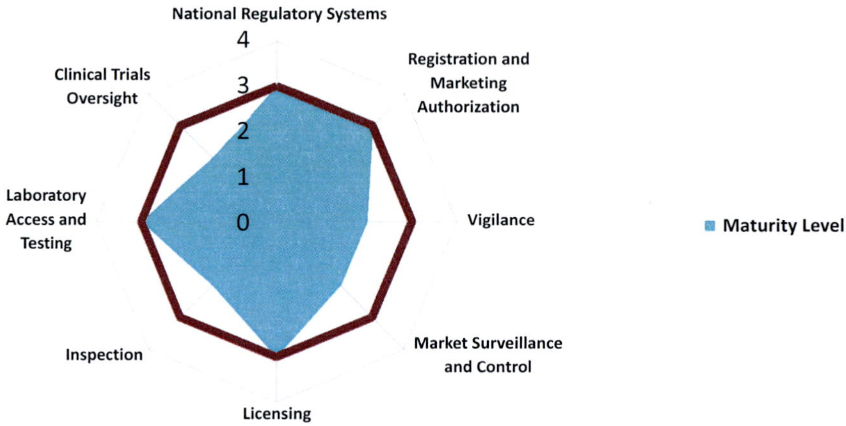

FIGURE 3-2 Spider web graph of a hypothetical agency's performance with the Global Benchmarking Tool.
SOURCE: Khadem, 2018.

Controls on the domestic food market are less predictable and harder to measure, described in *The Safe Food Imperative* as "sporadic and reactive, coming in the wake of major outbreaks of foodborne disease or food adulteration scandals" (Jaffee et al., 2019). In some ways, this makes the benchmarking process even more valuable, as the assessment can motivate investment in the food control system. The challenge of using benchmarking to this end is that there is no comprehensive, publicly available, standardized assessment tool relevant to low- and middle-income countries (Jaffee et al., 2019). *The Safe Food Imperative* commented on this problem, noting that, while detailed assessments of the systems have been done in many low- and middle-income countries, the findings, sometimes even the criteria assessed, are sensitive and not shared, "perhaps because of concerns about how the media or public would react to documented shortcomings" (Jaffee et al., 2019). Assessments of regulatory systems are sensitive, but this committee believes openness about the results is the best course of action. Furthermore, because food safety touches on many different fields, there are a variety of benchmarking tools that touch on different aspects of food safety. A comprehensive food safety benchmark analogous to that provided by the WHO Global Benchmarking Tool is desirable, and may be best approximated by the WHO and the FAO Food Control System Assessment Tool.

The Food Control System Assessment Tool

The WHO and the FAO Food Control System Assessment Tool can provide a useful benchmark for regulatory competence (FAO, 2019). The contents of this tool share many similarities with the Global Benchmarking Tool, including an emphasis on continuous improvement, assessment of key functions, and a final rating for the strength of the system (though this is not a rating for the agency or agencies involved) (Caipo, 2019; FAO and WHO, 2019b).

The Food Control System Assessment Tool was developed in 2014, building off publicly available assessment tools from the Inter-American Institute for Cooperation on Agriculture, the World Organisation for Animal Health, and the International Plant Protection Convention (FAO, 2014; FAO and WHO, 2019b). Figure 3-3 shows the four dimensions assessed in the evaluation (inputs and resources, control functions, interaction with stakeholders, science and knowledge base and continuous improvement), as well as the ways these dimensions are subdivided and the competencies assessed. Part of the process relies on self-assessment from people working in the regulatory agency, though assessors from the WHO, the FAO, or both will facilitate the process (Caipo, 2019). As with the Global Benchmarking Tool, scores on the WHO and the FAO food control assessment are meant to help regulators identify weaknesses and develop plans for improvement (FAO, 2019).

The Food Control System Assessment has only been publicly available since July 2019 (FAO and WHO, 2019a). Reports from as early as 2014 indicate that it was pilot tested in the Gambia, Indonesia, Iran, Malawi, Moldova, Morocco, Sierra Leone, Zambia, and Zimbabwe; results of these assessments are confidential, and sharing them is at the discretion of the participating country (FAO, 2014; STDF, n.d.b).[3] Coverage of a recent assessment in Indonesia, for example, commented on relative strengths in risk analysis but problems integrating information across different food safety agencies (TEMPO.CO, 2018). Like the Global Benchmarking Tool, the assessment is designed to produce a clear list of priorities and a strategy for improvement, and to give countries a baseline from which to monitor their progress (STDF, n.d.b). This exercise should, in turn, "help governments direct and integrate national investment with donor assistance" (STDF, n.d.b). Repeating the processes on a predictable timeline, every 5 years, for example, can help countries monitor their progress and identify new priorities for improvement.

[3] This text has changed since prepublication release of the report.

DIMENSIONS	SUBDIMENSIONS	SYSTEM COMPETENCIES
A INPUTS AND RESOURCES	A.1 POLICY AND LEGAL FRAMEWORKS	**A.1.1** Policy and legal drafting process
		A.1.2 Institutional framework
		A.1.3 Elements for food control legislation
	A.2 INFRASTRUCTURE AND FINANCE	**A.2.1** Financial resources
		A.2.2 Infrastructure and equipment
		A.2.3 Analytical resources
	A.3 HUMAN RESOURCES	**A.3.1** Qualification of personnel
		A.3.2 Capacity development of personnel
		A.3.3 Staff management and staff motivation
B CONTROL FUNCTIONS	B.1 ROUTINE CONTROL ACTIVITIES OVER FOOD PRODUCTS	**B.1.1** Domestic controls
		B.1.2 Import controls
		B.1.3 Export controls
	B.2 MONITORING, SURVEILLANCE, AND RESPONSE FUNCTIONS	**B.2.1** Monitoring programs in relation to the food chain
		B.2.2 Foodborne disease surveillance
		B.2.3 Management of food safety emergencies
C INTERACTIONS WITH STAKEHOLDERS	C.1 DOMESTIC STAKEHOLDERS	**C.1.1** Relationships between competent authorities and private sector regarding training needs
		C.1.2 Information flows and integration of business operators into risk management
		C.1.3 Communication flows and involvement with consumers
	C.2 INTERNATIONAL STAKEHOLDERS	**C.2.1** Interactions among competent authorities at international level
		C.2.2 Engagement of competent authorities into international organizations
D SCIENCE OR KNOWLEDGE BASE AND CONTINUOUS IMPROVEMENT	D.1 EVIDENCE AND RISK BASE	**D.1.1** Access of competent authorities to updated scientific and technical information
		D.1.2 Capacity to collect and analyze data for risk analysis purposes
		D.1.3 Knowledge and use by competent authorities of risk analysis framework
	D.2 CONTINUOUS IMPROVEMENT	**D.2.1** Performance monitoring of competent authorities and continuous improvement
		D.2.2 Mechanism to ensure consideration of newest scientific and technical information for food control

FIGURE 3-3 Structure of the Food Control Assessment Tool.
SOURCE: FAO and WHO, 2019b.

Other Food System Evaluations

One advantage of the WHO and the FAO Food Control System Assessment Tool is that it considers the full food safety system in a country. Other evaluations serve similar purposes for parts of the system. Assessment of animal or plant health can, when taken together, give a good picture of the food controls in a country.

The World Organisation for Animal Health Performance of Veterinary Systems Tool

In 2007 the World Organisation for Animal Health (known by the historical acronym OIE) released its Performance of Veterinary Services Pathway (OIE, 2017). Now in its sixth edition, the tool is published online (OIE, 2019). Though not a total food system assessment, the tool assesses veterinary services and health, which are relevant to the safety of high-risk, animal-source foods (Jaffee et al., 2019). Like other benchmarking assessments it brings external assessors to a country; the assessors evaluate the system, identify key gaps, and return for follow-up evaluations (Jaffee et al., 2019). (Figure 3-4 presents the steps in the evaluation cycle.) The gap analysis is organized according to relevant competencies in trade, animal health, veterinary public health, veterinary laboratories, and management and regulatory services (OIE, n.d.-b). It also facilitates the calculation on an annual budget and a separate budget for exceptional expenses (OIE, n.d.-b).

The OIE tool positions veterinary services as a global public good, necessary for both social and economic well-being (OIE, 2019). Final assessments are not public documents, though a growing list of countries has authorized the OIE to publish their gap analyses (Jaffee et al., 2019; OIE, n.d.-a). Development partners may also have access to the assessments, as the World Bank did, reporting on some aggregate information in the 2019 *The Safe Food Imperative* (Jaffee et al., 2019). Their analysis concluded that, across low- and middle-income countries, surveillance for disease and food safety is deficient, and traceability is negligible (Jaffee et al., 2019). As Figure 3-5 indicates, a large share of upper-middle-income countries perform adequately in key functions but still have strong capacity in only a minority of areas (Jaffee et al., 2019).

The International Plant Protection Convention's Phytosanitary Capacity Evaluation

The International Plant Protection Convention (a treaty overseen by the FAO) has a plant health evaluation called the Phytosanitary Capacity Evaluation Tool that may be analogous to the OIE tool. This evaluation differs from the FAO and the OIE assessments discussed previously in that,

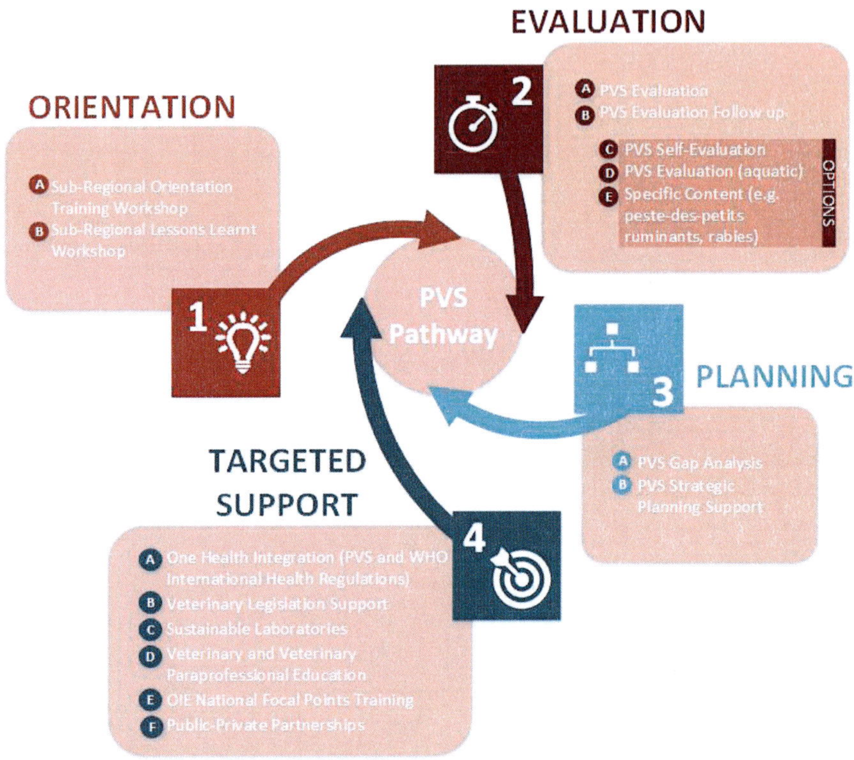

FIGURE 3-4 The OIE Performance of Veterinary Services Pathway.
SOURCE: OIE, 2019.

although it involves an external facilitator, the process and substance of the evaluation are left largely to the participating country, even in determining what pieces of the national plant health system to evaluate (FAO, 2017a). As with the other assessments, the results are confidential. The items assessed are also not public, out of concern that applying the evaluation without proper facilitation would lead to invalid conclusions (FAO, 2017a). Broadly speaking, the tool has 13 modules, each one dealing with a different aspect of a national plant health system, including its legislative protections; resources; surveillance and reporting capacity; import regulatory system; and export, re-export, and transit systems (FAO, 2017a).

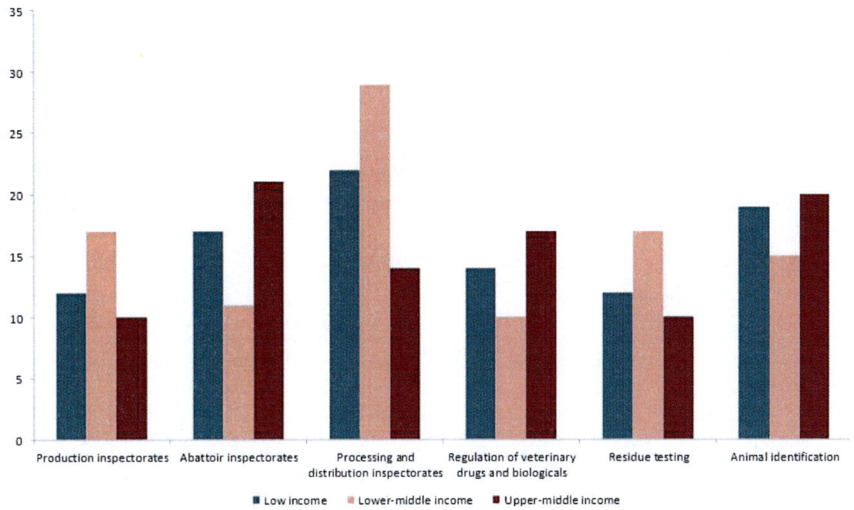

FIGURE 3-5 Animal product safety capacity, performance of veterinary services assessment in 93 countries.
SOURCE: Jaffee et al., 2019.

Assessment Results and Planning

The results of benchmarking assessments, be they those discussed in this chapter or others, are valuable to many stakeholders. First, they give the regulatory agencies, and the citizens to whom they are accountable, an idea of how well the system works. These results also allow for comparison between regulatory authorities. Such comparison can be especially useful for countries pursuing work sharing. By giving a common set of criteria and functions to aim for, benchmarking can facilitate harmonization (Ndomondo-Sigonda et al., 2017). The results also send a signal about an agency's ability to ensure quality food and drugs for domestic and international use.

In 2018, about a quarter of WHO member states had medicines regulatory authorities functioning at level three or higher (Khadem, 2018). Roughly the same proportion were at level two; half were at level one (Khadem, 2018). Less is known about the results of various food control assessment tools. Still, a review of FAO assessments in South and Southeast Asia identified common problems, including lack of clarity on which standards are voluntary and which are mandatory; laboratories not being accredited; poor coordination and overlapping mandates among food regulatory agencies; laws and processes not made with attention to risk; and a lack of reliable data (Jaffee et al., 2019).

Countries need to know how their regulatory systems are performing relative to other countries' agencies and over time. But simply measuring performance will not encourage progress in itself. Benchmarking should also fit into a larger institutional development plan. The assessment is the first step; strengths and weaknesses identified in this assessment inform the next step: drafting of an institutional development plan. This is a short-term (roughly 5-year) strategy that breaks down the tasks needed for an agency into specific steps and priorities. This plan should set out terms for monitoring and for corrective actions when targets are not met on time.

The results of the benchmarking assessment, as well as the budget and the institutional development plans they inform, should then be shared with a coalition of interested partners, including both public- and private-sector partners who can help with capacity building. The WHO has pilot projects using a coalition model to support regulatory agencies in Bangladesh and in sub-Saharan Africa (WHO, 2019a,d). The weaknesses identified in the assessment are the areas donors can target their support. For example, if a country was short of meeting the Global Benchmarking Tool's level three cut point in inspection and vigilance, then those functions would be the target of donor funding.

Recommendation 3-1: Development partners, including multilateral and bilateral donors and private philanthropic organizations, should encourage countries' participation in regulatory benchmarking assessments, the development of institutional development plans, and reports on progress against those plans. To this end, assistance should be targeted to priorities identified in benchmarking assessments and the related institutional development plans.

Benchmarking of regulatory systems is a valuable process in itself. It brings external assessors to a system and gives the agency's leaders a time to reflect on priorities and think strategically about improvement. The results of the assessment facilitate harmonization and allow for comparison among agencies and within the same agency over time. The tools also translate the daunting and sometimes vague concept of regulatory performance into concrete tasks, and provide for regular checks on progress (Roth et al., 2018a). Benchmarking also has a valuable self-assessment component. The international team responsible for the Global Benchmarking Tool evaluation also facilitates the participating agency's staff to make institutional development plans (Branigan, 2019).

None of these benefits can be realized, however, unless countries choose to participate in the assessment. This is precisely why an incentive in the form of donor assistance would be valuable. Donors can encourage participation by tying their support to the agency's institutional development plan. This strategy would magnify the value of the donor contribution, by using it to influence recipient countries to go through a benchmarking assessment. It would also help ensure that the aid provided is in line with local priorities. The point of the institutional development plan, after all, is to identify priority actions that can improve the agency in the next 5 years. Incorporating the results of the benchmarking assessment into a concrete and time-bound plan can also help drive progress, raising the visibility of the regulatory agency within government (Kaddu et al., 2018). Ministers of health and agriculture have many competing priorities, after all. Measurement, assessment, and re-assessment of regulatory gaps can help keep up momentum for investing in regulatory systems even in the face of other demands.

An additional and desirable level of accountability would come from making the results of the assessment public, something none of the assessments require. The committee recognizes the reasons why agencies might resist disclosing their results. Food and medicines regulation can be highly sensitive topics, and agencies might have reasonable concerns about how any shortcomings would be perceived in the press (Jaffee et al., 2019). The organizations conducting the benchmarking assessment, for their part, cannot compel sovereign governments to share information with the public. However, the global expectation of transparency—and support from key donors—could create significant pressure on governments to do so.

A strong argument for making benchmarking assessments public is that transparency can influence policy (Hale and Held, 2011). The process can help governments develop functioning, integrated regulatory systems that benefit their citizens and consumers around the world (Jaffee et al., 2019). Donors can use their influence to encourage this process. For example, countries that may resist sharing their results might be persuaded to allow partial public access or access to certain intermediaries. Development partners such as the World Bank have selective access to the OIE veterinary assessments, for example, as this information can inform the Bank's investments in a country (Jaffee et al., 2019). In the same way, the committee envisions donors, acting individually or as a coalition, using the gaps identified through benchmarking and the related institutional development plans as a roadmap for their support. Working together toward progress on the institutional development plans also gives donors a chance to encourage their host country counterparts to publicize progress and eventually to make results public.

It is in the best interest of all development partners that regulatory systems in low- and middle-income countries perform better. Investing in these institutions is a worthy priority for donors and one entirely in line with principles of aid effectiveness. It would also contribute to more vigorous local markets in low- and middle-income countries, something that would benefit everyone.

Considerations in Procurement

The Paris Declaration emphasis on untying of aid was meant to improve efficiency and value for money (Clay et al., 2009). The more recent move toward universal coverage makes these concerns even more pressing. Countries, including those middle-income countries transitioning away from multilateral funding, are, because of universal coverage, now responsible for the purchase of more and varied types of medicines (Silverman et al., 2019; Tatay and Torreele, 2019; Wagner et al., 2014).

Procurement poses many challenges for buyers in low- and middle-income countries. Regulatory hurdles, such as the process required for registration in a country, can make procurement less efficient (Silverman et al., 2019). Registering more and different types of medicines puts a burden on the regulatory agency, often far exceeding its capacity in low- and middle-income countries (Roth et al., 2018a).

Modern manufacturing can also make it difficult to weigh the essential procurement question of value for money. As Figure 3-6 shows, some parts of the world (South Asia for instance) have considerable local manufacturing, while most medical products used in sub-Saharan Africa are imported (Silverman et al., 2019). Ensuring quality for imported products is challenging for any regulatory agency, and especially so for ones with fewer resources.

As the previous chapter explained, the WHO Prequalification Program provides assessment, inspection, and ongoing re-inspection of manufacturers and consistency testing and quality control for certain vaccines, medicines, and other medical products. As such, it can be a boon to procurement agencies, acting as a proxy regulatory approval, something especially valuable in managing the combination of limited regulatory capacity and foreign suppliers. To be clear, however, the WHO does *not* act as a supra-national regulatory agency through prequalification (Stahl, 2013). Prequalification does not provide the key regulatory responsibility of market authorization, though some countries may use it for that purpose (Stahl, 2013).

The Prequalification Program is also one of the best tools for building capacity in medicines regulation. Every step of the prequalification assessment, including dossier review and site inspections, is conducted by teams made up of WHO staff, regulators from advanced agencies, and regulators from the countries where the prequalified products will be used (WHO, n.d.-a). This allows for hands-on training by conducting the reviews, a valuable exercise for the regulators involved. Furthermore, regulators in the

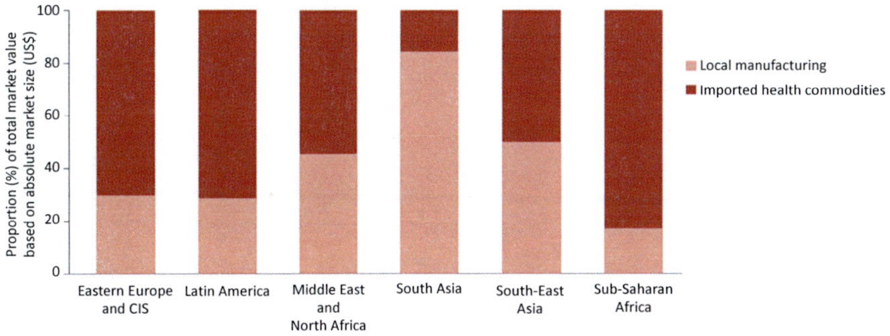

FIGURE 3-6 Average proportion of local manufacturing and importation of medicines and vaccines.
NOTE: CIS = Commonwealth of Independent States.
SOURCE: Silverman et al., 2019.

home country of the manufacturer applying for prequalification can join prequalification inspections, even if they are not part of the assessment team (Stahl, 2013). Regulators from developing countries can also participate in a three-month rotating position at WHO headquarters to get experience of prequalification and deeper knowledge of other areas that influence medicines regulation ('t Hoen et al., 2014).

Capacity building also extends to WHO's prequalification of quality control labs, which provides technical assistance and management audits to help ensure the labs can operate to international standards (WHO, n.d.-e). The program also has been found to have positive spillover effects on manufacturing, with production lines for both prequalified and non-prequalified products benefiting from manufacturers' participation in the program (WHO, 2019b).

WHO prequalification started in 1987 as a check on the quality of vaccines procured through UNICEF or other UN agencies (Dellepiane and Wood, 2015; WHO, 2013). In 2001 the program expanded to include medicines for HIV procured through UNAIDS and other UN agencies; it quickly expanded to include treatments for tuberculosis and malaria (Stahl, 2013). Today about 1,700 products have prequalification, including treatments for hepatitis and diarrheal disease. Some neglected tropical diseases are included in prequalification, as are various vector control products, diagnostic kits, immunization devices, and reproductive health products (WHO, 2019b). By 2019 estimates, the Prequalification Program enables a market of about $3.5 billion annually, allowing an additional 340–400 million people to access treatment they might not otherwise have had (WHO, 2019b, n.d.-d).

As of late 2019, there were 553 medicines on the WHO prequalified list, the vast majority treatments for HIV, tuberculosis, or malaria (WHO, n.d.-b). The types of products listed for prequalification reflect the demand of the program's main clients: UN agencies, the Global Fund, and large donors. There is room to make the program more useful to other large buyers of medical products, including low- and middle-income country governments and the private businesses that do a great deal of procurement in those countries (Silverman et al., 2019). To this end, the *Lancet* Commission on Essential Medicines recommended the expansion of WHO prequalification to include more medicines (Wirtz et al., 2017). The most recent meeting of the International Conference of Drug Regulatory Authorities called for the same, citing the program's ability to improve access to quality-assured medicines, and its role in meeting the increasing demands of universal coverage (ICDRA, 2018). If given the option of buying from prequalified suppliers, large procurement agencies could reliably use their purchasing power to promote medicines quality.

Recommendation 3-2: The World Health Organization should expand prequalification to include treatments for cancer, diabetes, and other diseases with a high global burden.

The WHO Prequalification Program provides a global public good. It also improves health, increasing the supply of good-quality, affordable medical products in low- and middle-income countries (Unitaid, n.d.). A larger list of reputable, quality-assured medicines would give procurement officers a tool to navigate an otherwise murky market. Expanding the list of prequalified products to be more in line with the burden of disease in aid recipient countries would also help countries ensure their medicines budgets are going to reliable products. As the move to universal coverage increases the burden on this budget, the question of value for money will be even more important. Ultimately, good procurement protects the population from the risk posed by poor quality medicines.

Prequalification is also a proven investment in building capacity for medicines regulation (Dellepiane and Wood, 2015; WHO, 2013). Through its design the program takes advantage of technical depth at advanced regulatory agencies (those benchmarked at level four or higher), without duplicating their work, though products approved by these agencies are given an abridged review in the prequalification process (Rägo, 2012). The Global Fund guidance on procurement also allows procurement of products approved for use by advanced regulatory agencies (The Global Fund, 2018).

Expanding WHO prequalification could also help ensure a vigorous market for quality-assured generics. Prequalified companies increase their chances of international procurement; they may also expand their local markets. This is a potential benefit; uncertain demand is difficult for honest manufacturers to manage. High variability impedes efficiency and scale; it also makes for higher transaction costs that are then passed along to consumers (Silverman et al., 2019). A 2019 assessment found that every dollar spent in running prequalification returns 30 to 40 times that amount in savings during procurement and by leveling the playing field to allow good manufacturers in low- and middle-income countries entry to international markets (WHO, 2019b).

In its 5-year plan to help build regulatory systems, the WHO cited strengthening and expansion of prequalification as a strategic priority (WHO, 2019a). To this end, the 5-year plan discussed ways to improve awareness of the program, especially the capacity building piece that regulators might not be aware of, and the spillover benefits to local manufacturing (WHO, 2019a). Regarding the expansion of the prequalification list, the 5-year plan highlighted in vitro diagnostics and vector control products (WHO, 2019a). The committee supports this plan and sees this recommendation as part of a global consensus on the value of the program (ICDRA, 2018; Wirtz et al., 2017). At the same time, it encourages WHO authorities to look beyond products associated with HIV, malaria, tuberculosis, and reproductive health. As of late 2019, only about 17 percent of products on the WHO Model Essential Medicines List have even one prequalified supplier.[4]

The choice of medicines and the order at which they are added to the program is a topic for further discussion. The information available in the Global Burden of Disease reports regarding both the prevalence and relative harm of different conditions would be part of this discussion (IHME, n.d.). Products for smaller but important markets, such as neglected diseases, should also be considered. There is also clear demand for any product where a third or more of the total market by volume is subject to global procurement. Medicines that present a particular challenge to regulators because of the complexity of manufacturing would also be good candidates ('t Hoen et al., 2014), as would anti-infectives since the risk of drug resistance makes the quality of these products a global public good.

Expansion of the prequalification program would improve access and reduce costs of whole families of important products (e.g., antidiabetics and cancer treatments). It would also have other helpful effects. The use of poor quality antimicrobials, for example, contributes to resistance, a problem of serious public health consequence around the world (IADB, 2017). Prequalification of those antimicrobials at high risk for quality problems,

[4] Percentage calculated from WHO, 2019c,e.

beta-lactams for example, might also be a strategy for reducing resistance (Fair and Tor, 2014; Kelesidis and Falagas, 2015).

One important feature of the Prequalification Program is its ongoing quality control efforts, including re-inspection, quality monitoring, field sampling and testing, and monitoring of quality control laboratories (WHO, n.d.-c). The expansion envisioned in this report would give considerable attention to these measures *taken after listing*. Such post-approval quality control is not emphasized as part of the expansion of prequalification described in the WHO's recent strategy document, although there is attention to building capacity for post-market surveillance in general (WHO, 2019a).

Critics of this strategy might maintain that prequalification was meant to be an interim solution as countries develop their regulatory and procurement systems (Dellepiane and Wood, 2015). Nevertheless, today the program fills an important void, not just in the assessment and quality control for certain drugs, but in capacity building for both regulators and manufacturers. Therefore, the committee concurs with the *Lancet* Commission on Essential Medicines, that more types of products be included in prequalification, "at least until ... the global generic market has developed sufficient capacity" to meet the increased demand universal coverage will bring (Wirtz et al., 2017).

The development of capacity is central to the Prequalification Program and to this recommendation. One aspect of capacity building is increasing ability—that of regulators, of manufacturers, of procurement programs—to operate well. WHO prequalification has, by design, considerable emphasis on this aspect of capacity building, as discussed earlier in this section. It is important to remember, however, that building capacity also refers to improving the total resources available for a job. For some agencies, this increase in capacity comes mainly from sharing information to avoid duplication of work; international harmonization and regulatory convergence (discussed later in this report) are tools to the same end. Prequalification of medicines provides a global public good, even beyond its staff development component. Expansion of the program would increase the public good and allow regulatory and procurement agencies to work more efficiently.

The committee recognizes that the products on the prequalification list to date are those procured by international agencies, whereas procurement of medicines for cancer and other chronic diseases are mostly domestic responsibilities. National procurement cannot command the same negotiating power as major donors placing pooled orders (Tatay and Torreele, 2019). At the same time, there is growing interest in helping countries respond to the challenges of noncommunicable diseases. The Defeat NCD Partnership, for example, is a group of governments; civil society; academic, philanthropic, and research organizations; private businesses; and multilaterals committed to fighting noncommunicable disease, especially in the 49 least developed countries (The Defeat-NCD Partnership, n.d.-a, n.d.-c). Its financing facility aims to help countries create fiscal space for related efforts, with additional donor funding, bonds, and other tools (The Defeat-NCD Partnership, n.d.-b). The donor initiative Resolve to Save Lives is similarly committed to expanding access to anti-hypertensives globally (Vital Strategies, n.d.). Some of these programs are still in early stages, and expanded prequalification might better position them to procure large orders as the Global Fund does.

Expanding prequalification also puts a burden on the WHO and other participants in the program. Some of that burden will come in the form of increased demand for expertise. Prequalification review depends on the contributed short-term expertise from regulators from advanced agencies[5] (WHO, n.d.-f). Expansion of prequalification will increase the demand for such service, meaning more regulators asking for time away from their routine duties. The FDA and other level four agencies may need to adjust their staffing projections to ensure they can do their part to meet this demand.

There is also a direct financial burden on the WHO. Manufacturers are charged user fees to participate in prequalification; before user fees were introduced (in 1999 for vaccines, 2008 for diagnostics, and 2013 for medicines) the only donors to the program were UNICEF, the Bill & Melinda Gates Foundation, and Unitaid (WHO, n.d.-h). In an effort to improve the program's sustainability, the WHO revised its fee structure in 2017 (WHO, n.d.-h). Under the new structure user fees are meant to cover about half of the program's operating costs, with fees waived for important products with small markets (WHO, n.d.-h). The use of fees to support prequalification also brings challenges, especially for products with small markets and for which the volume under global procurement is small.

Ideally, this report and the wider consensus about global public goods of which it is a part, would encourage the United States and other rich countries to pay their full assessed contributions to the WHO, thereby alleviating some of the financial strain of this recommendation. Advanced regulatory agencies (those benchmarked at WHO level four) also have a role in increasing resources for prequalification. Staff from these agencies support prequalification by taking part in the dossier reviews and inspections. As much as possible, they should advocate for more support for it from their agencies and from their countries' aid organizations.

[5] Those performing at level four or higher on the Global Benchmarking Tool assessment.

Data and Standards

Expanding WHO prequalification and benchmarking regulatory systems both serve the goal of improving efficiency and access to good-quality products, something of crucial importance to under-resourced agencies. These recommendations, if implemented, could bring new products into low- and middle-income country markets, new opportunities for capacity building, and a new, impartial analysis of the regulatory system. There are also ways to improve product safety by making better use of some of the information already collected.

The routine operations of governments, businesses, and nonprofits today produce a great deal of information (Marvin et al., 2016). Unlocking the potential in this information, particularly its potential for public health, remains a challenge, however. Especially in low- and middle-income countries, the systems and skills needed to manage data exceed local capacity (Mathauer et al., 2017). There can also be obstacles in the form of an organizational culture that does not encourage sharing, or even generating, information (Mathauer et al., 2017).

Such reticence is understandable. There is a cost to disclosing information, both directly, in terms of staff time or technical upgrades, and indirectly. Data sharing can be technically difficult because different organizations have different ways of collecting and managing the same or similar information; their data systems are not likely to be interoperable without deliberate attention (Gascó et al., 2018). The decision to share data requires participants to overcome the fear that information could be used against them (Gascó et al., 2018).

At the same time, large datasets can be useful to regulators. The post-market surveillance of medicines, for example, could be made easier by using the information in electronic medical records or the copious, unreported data collected in clinical trials (IRPCV, 2018; Ross, 2014). Making use of these data can be difficult, though. Advanced regulatory authorities are struggling with adjustments to their legal authority and guidelines brought about by so-called big data (EMA, 2019; Martin, 2017).

The idea of big data is applied to food safety less frequently, partly because the information, while just as vast, is scattered among more and disparate sources (Marvin et al., 2016). Simply identifying and linking relevant information from across these sources presents a challenge (Marvin et al., 2016). The technology exists to trace food through the supply chain, with tremendous potential to control foodborne disease. For farmers, especially small farmers in low- and middle-income countries, access and ability to use powerful handheld technology for data collection can be a barrier to traceability, though the best incentives to encourage data collection and sharing at the level of the small farmer are not necessarily clear (Gascó et al., 2018).

Sharing data could change the way regulators work with their counterparts in other countries (EMA, 2019). Regulatory inspections, for example, are a considerable staff burden on both regulators and industry (Rönninger et al., 2017). There is wide consensus that collaboration and joint inspection help control this burden (FDA, 2018d; ICDRA, 2016; IOM, 2012a; WHO, 2012). Similar data standards could help translate this and other principles of regulatory cooperation into action.

Box 3-1 explains what data standards are and why they are important. Common rules on how to collect and store data help industry manage risks (Davidson, 2016). Data standards are also the foundation of the regulatory agency's public health risk ranking. The development of tools to rank and assess risks is central to a risk-based regulatory system (IOM and NRC, 2010). Information about risks also facilitates work sharing among regulators, a topic discussed more in Chapter 5.

When resources are scarce, the imperative to make good use of what is available increases. For regulatory agencies this means facilitating the sharing of data among different government agencies and industry. Sharing data means organizing a vast amount of information. There are tradeoffs when collecting such information, between accuracy, ease and speed of collection, and the expense of the undertaking (Martin, 2017). Donor funding could minimize the technical obstacles and expense of data sharing, helping to tip the balance of tradeoffs in favor of openness.

Recommendation 3-3: Development partners, including multilateral and bilateral donors and private philanthropic organizations, should support countries and regional organizations in pursuing greater collaboration for regulating food and medical products. This collaboration can include harmonization and mutual recognition of data or standards, equivalence agreements, and regulatory reliance.

Information sharing "is key to reaping the public value from all kinds of data" (Gascó et al., 2018). Particularly in food safety, no one organization has enough information to ensure traceability through the supply chain (Susha et al., 2019). Data sharing also produces a public good. The information generated can inform public policy and risk-to-benefit analysis; it can be used to answer valuable research questions (Gascó et al., 2018). Box 3-2 describes one such data-sharing program, the U.S. Department of Agriculture (USDA) Global Branded Food Products Database.

The technical costs of data sharing, while by no means the only barrier, are a serious obstacle to regulatory collaboration. By providing an interoperable infrastructure and data standards, donors could help overcome the initial cost of data sharing, magnifying the value of their contribution.

BOX 3-1
What Are Data Standards?

Data standards are rules by which datasets are described and recorded. To share, exchange, and understand data, the format and meaning must be standardized in a way that can be clearly understood.

Data standardization allows us to easily share and reuse a dataset. For example, when you buy batteries you need not worry about which brand of batteries you buy: an AA battery from any brand will fit into an AA space.

The value of data is realized more easily when users need to do as little work as possible to clean or reformat the data for their needs. Data standards are what enable us to achieve this.

SOURCE: FSA, 2019.

Sharing information also depends on strong relationships among collaborators (Gascó et al., 2018). Providing data standards and a common platform could also help build trust among regulators and advance the long-term goal of regulatory harmonization.

THE ROLE OF COMMERCE

The World Trade Organization (WTO) describes trade as, "an engine for inclusive economic growth and poverty reduction" and a force for sustainable development (UN, n.d.). Trade in medical products, and especially in food, can be important in low- and middle-income countries where the domestic market alone cannot stimulate industry or support manufacturing at a sufficient scale to be efficient (Elliott, 2019). In such cases, trade has the potential to improve both livelihoods and the quality of products in the market.

Trade associations have an interest in strong, fair regulatory systems for products their members produce. They can spur interest in strengthening these systems. In Colombia, for example, political interest in free trade agreements translated into increased appropriations to the Invima (the food and drug regulatory agency) starting around 2012 (Guzman, 2019). In 2016, WHO benchmarking established Invima at level four, thereby increasing the market for Colombian products around Latin America (Guzman, 2019). As the former agency head explained, "Invima, as a reference agency of the Americas, is now leading the government efforts to open new

BOX 3-2
The U.S. Department of Agriculture (USDA) Global Branded Food Products Database

The USDA Global Branded Food Products Database provides nutrition information and ingredients from product labels. Launched in September 2016, the database runs as a public–private partnership that includes the USDA, International Life Sciences Institute (ILSI) North America (a science nonprofit concerned with food and nutrition), the U.S. division of the global information standards organization GS1, WorldSync (a technology services company), the University of Maryland's Joint Institute for Food Safety and Applied Nutrition, and the Label Insight software service. The USDA's National Agricultural Library hosts and maintains the data for public use, including education, research, and food regulatory efforts.

The database gives the public access to a great deal of nutritional information. It can instantly link serving size and nutrient content with information on diet and on dietary recommendations, thereby enriching the USDA's efforts to understand population nutrition and the composition of the food supply, essential data for setting food and agriculture policy. Its inclusion of branded foods complements information in the older USDA FoodData Central database.

Participation in the program is voluntary but requires submission of all information about a set of "mandatory attributes," such as product description, serving size, servings per package, nutrition label information, ingredients, and date of the most current formulation. Participants can submit these data through one of two secure methods: the USDA's Label Insight portal, or, for GS1 clients, via synchronizing product information in the GS1 system.

As of August 2019, the USDA Global Branded Food Products Database included over 247,000 products. And, because all entries are archived, information on changes in food composition over time is also easily tracked. The speed at which data can be accessed, especially compared to methods such as biochemical analysis, is a clear advantage. The database also greatly reduces the cost of data collection and ensures that data are stored in a common, usable format. Interest in the database is global, with tracked usage in Canada, the United Kingdom, India, Mexico, Spain, Brazil, Germany, and Italy. The partnership's organizers hope to increase the number of private label food items in the database and to add restaurant foods and imported foods.

SOURCES: Avant, 2018; GS1 US, 2016; ILSI, n.d.; Kretser et al., 2017; Starke-Reed, 2017.

markets for products manufactured in Colombia and improve the country's competitiveness" (Pharma Boardroom, 2017).

At the same time, movement of food and drugs across borders can aggravate the information asymmetry already inherent in these markets. Inspection and assessment from an independent party can help correct this imbalance, as the WHO Prequalification Program does. Food production, in contrast to medicines, has far more sprawling and complicated supply chains, with multiple, legitimate markets in the same places. As the previous chapter discussed, quality certifications from external third parties are important in food and agriculture, but the balance of benefits and harms, especially to small producers in poor countries, is not always clear (Henson and Humphrey, 2010).

The ability of food producers to comply with international standards, be they Codex standards or the sometimes more exacting private ones, can be used as a proxy indicator of the capacity in a country for managing safety and quality (Jaffee et al., 2019). This capacity does not necessarily permeate the domestic market, however. Certain conditions encourage so-called positive spillovers: when the exported food is also widely consumed locally, for example, or when its production is widespread and not consolidated, when the leading processing companies produce for both domestic and export markets, and when modern retail is common and well developed (STDF, n.d.a). These conditions are not often met in low- or middle-income countries.

Therefore, despite the potential for international food standards to improve food safety, evidence supporting such effects is limited and mixed, probably because the export and domestic food markets in low- and middle-income countries are fairly segregated (Jaffee et al., 2019; STDF, n.d.a). On one hand, some research has found that products failing to meet standards for supermarkets or chain retail are dumped to informal markets (Roesel et al., 2014). The quality of food in informal markets is a concern, since they are the main source of animal-source foods for people in Africa and Asia (Grace et al., 2014). They are also crucial to the economy of low- and middle-income countries. Informal, international trade employs between 20 and 70 percent of sub-Saharan Africa, disproportionately women (FAO, 2017b).

The challenge remains to encourage producers to meet international standards, and to do so in a way that benefits all consumers. Technical assistance can be valuable, and may encourage broad changes to production, such as better farm management (Unnevehr and Ronchi, 2014). But it is difficult to say how much technical assistance for meeting standards helps producers in low- and middle-income countries because so much depends on prevailing market conditions, which can change abruptly (Unnevehr and Ronchi, 2014). Compliance with international standards has a cost, though the cost can be regained through wider market access (Unnevehr and Ronchi, 2014).

Investing in Safety and Quality

Regulatory enforcement is one means to improve products, but the regulator's power to change manufacturing practices is limited if the market is not supporting standards. A complete strategy for global action to improve food safety and drug quality must consider the role of market incentives. Large market actors can use their influence to raise product standards. The previous chapter discussed the role of supermarket chains to compel their suppliers to meet third-party standards; the power of large procurement agencies on the medicines market is similar. Market incentives can also be used to encourage producers to invest in quality for the domestic market, as in the Twiga Foods example discussed in Box 3-3.

Investing in quality brings new markets and other opportunities to grow businesses; it can even improve cost-efficiency. The switch from batch processing to continuous manufacturing, for example, allows for a greater volume produced and carries fewer opportunities for contamination (Chatterjee, 2012; Comerford, 2018). Such benefits are not always clear to the people in a position to change business practices. Even when they are, the cost of the capital available from local banks and capital markets in low- and middle-income countries may be too high to make the investment viable (Papadavid, 2017).

Banks in emerging markets usually have especially limited products available to small- and medium-sized businesses, because the credit assessment and costs of making the loan drive up its cost (Abraham and Schmukler, 2017; Abuka et al., 2019; GFSI, 2018). As a result, the small- and medium-sized business owners in developing economies cite access to capital as one of their biggest obstacles (IFC, n.d.-b).

Nevertheless, the private sector in low- and middle-income countries is growing. Private financing to sub-Saharan Africa, for example, has grown in the last decade, but most of this growth has been directed to extractive industries, with two countries (Nigeria and Ethiopia) receiving about two-thirds of all private-sector financing in the region (Tyson, 2017). Only about 12 percent of foreign investment in sub-Saharan Africa is for manufacturing and 2 percent for agriculture (Tyson, 2017). This is unfortunate, as investments in agribusiness and manufacturing have some of the best effects on poverty reduction (Karim and Buckley, 2015). In general, investments in agribusiness and infrastructure have been catalytic in low- and lower-middle-income countries, whereas support for industry and infrastructure has benefited the upper-middle-income countries the most (Massa, 2011).

BOX 3-3
Twiga Foods

Market access has traditionally been a problem for small farmers in Africa. Since traveling to the wholesale market takes time away from work and may require vehicles they do not have, farmers have long relied on brokers to take their products to market. The brokers' fees detract from their profits and contribute to a lack of transparency in the market. Vendors also spend time and money traveling to wholesale markets and transporting produce to their stalls, usually without refrigeration. At Twiga collection centers farmers can meet with agronomists to discuss strategies to improve crop yields; they can also access tailored financial services.

Twiga Foods is a Kenyan firm that uses mobile phones to connect small farmers to vendors. This removes several costly intermediary steps in the distribution chain, thereby allowing better prices for both the farmers selling produce and the vendors buying it. Twiga also manages a direct-to-retail distribution system, complete with a refrigerated distribution center, 12 collection centers, and a fleet of distribution trucks. Use of the fast and modern distribution system has reduced post-harvest losses by about 25 percentage points.

Twiga Foods' expansion in 2018 and 2019 was financed in part by $10.3 million from the International Finance Corporation. About 13,000 farmers and 10,000 vendors now use the Twiga system and, as part of their expansion, the company is now training farmers, processors, and vendors in good agricultural practices and quality certification for the Kenyan market.

SOURCES: FSN, 2019; IFC, 2018; Omondi, 2019.

Development banks and bilateral development finance organizations can lower the cost of equity and make investments in quality more profitable for businesses in low- and middle-income countries. The organizations may do this through concessional financing, meaning loans with considerably more generous terms (in interest or repayment periods or both) than the market would offer (OECD, 2003). They also provide advisory services to companies regarding how to meet international best practices, and how to enter new markets, attract investors, and improve performance (IFC, n.d.-a). It is important to note that capital supplied through development finance is additional to what the market would otherwise supply (FMO, 2016, 2018). And World Bank research has found that, as countries' incomes increase, the private sector may be able to supply more capital, making their advisory services and support for development of global public goods more prominent (WBG, 2018).There is a role for both types of products in making improvements to agribusiness and medicines manufacturing in low- and middle-income countries.

Recommendation 3-4: Development finance institutions such as the United States International Development Finance Corporation, the International Finance Corporation (IFC), the UK CDC Group, and the European development finance banks should create vehicles to finance producers, distributors, and retailers in low-and middle-income countries interested in meeting regulatory standards. This would involve advisory services and, when appropriate, concessional financing.

Development banks and bilateral development finance organizations increasingly emphasize how well their investments contribute to the poverty reduction, social welfare, and the Sustainable Development Goals (FMO, 2016; Massa, 2011). Investing in quality manufacturing of essential medicines and the safe production of food is in line with these goals and is becoming more common. Box 3-3 describes an IFC program in Kenya to increase farmers' access to markets. The IFC also offers short-term working capital to food producers certified through the Global Food Safety Initiative as part of its programming to improve food safety and efficient production (GFSI, 2018). Through its MedAccess program, CDC Group, the British development finance agency has lowered the risk to market entry for suppliers of medical products in South Asia and sub-Saharan Africa (CDC Group, n.d.). MedAccess gives suppliers of certain high-quality medical products a safety net as they introduce new products in their markets, by contracting maximum prices in return for guaranteed sales; if actual sales fall short of the set threshold, MedAccess pays the supplier the difference (MedAccess, n.d.). The committee commends such innovative strategies and encourages wider user of investment vehicles to improve medicines and food safety in low- and middle-income countries. These investments should be evaluated to assess their contributions to product safety and quality; results of such evaluations could be used to make future investment programs more efficient.

This recommendation is concerned with both the advisory services and the lending functions of development finance. First, the organizations can help producers, distributors, and retailers along the supply chain identify future revenue and growth opportunities that could be realized by internalizing higher quality standards. When analysis of future revenue does not favor the change to higher standards, concessionary finance could adjust that calculation.

Tools for Quality Assurance

There are also global companies that are active in quality testing, but are not necessarily expanding in low- and middle-income countries. Food safety testing for pathogens and chemical substances is projected to grow rapidly in Asia over the next 5 years (Global Industry Analysts, 2019), though expansion potential in Africa and Latin America is less clear. Investing in these companies' expansion into underserved markets could also be a role for development finance.

Quality verification along the supply chain is essential for manufacturers monitoring their processes and outputs; it can also be important further down the supply chain. The assigning of unique identifiers at every step in the food distribution system is essential for traceability (Fernandez, 2019). Barcode serialization in medicines serves a similar goal (Rasheed et al., 2018). Nevertheless, the costs of such measures can be prohibitive for manufacturers, processors, and distributors in low- and middle-income countries (Pisa and McCurdy, 2019).

There are also ways to verify products already in circulation, often at point of entry or point of use (Lalani et al., 2017). Such testing is not a substitute for regulatory checks, or for a full quality assurance process in manufacturing, but is important to the system. In countries with weak regulatory capacity, screening technologies have a complementary role in improving quality (Jahnke, 2018; Lalani et al., 2017). They also provide regulators with much-needed tools for monitoring and can reduce the burden on the central testing laboratories (Roth et al., 2018b). Results from rapid screening assessments can also give regulators a sense of the types of problems common in their markets (Roth et al., 2018b).

Measuring the burden of falsified and substandard medicines, for example, depends on an analytical workflow that can be challenging in low- and middle-income countries (Fernandez et al., 2011). Screening technologies can help manage this workflow. The U.S. Food and Drug Administration's (FDA's) Counterfeit Detection devices, which can be used to compare the fluorescence of tablets, coating, packaging, food, or other regulated products to a verified sample, are one example of useful screening technologies (Batson et al., 2016; Platek et al., 2016). A European Commission consortium recently developed a handheld scanner that can detect falsified products using radiofrequency (Chen et al., 2016). Other technologies depend on physical, chemical, and microbiological analysis (Ellis et al., 2015; IOM, 2013; Kovacs et al., 2014).

The uptake of these tools at scale in low- and middle-income countries has been limited, however (Nayyar et al., 2015). A recent survey of regulators, manufacturers, distributors, and pharmacists in ten mostly low- or middle-income countries identified, "a technology gap in the development of affordable, easy to use, and precise screening technologies" (Roth et al., 2018b). The main reasons for this gap include the cost of training to use new technological tools, the cost of equipment and consumable materials, the management of supplies and reagents, and information about the relative strengths and weaknesses of the different methods (Roth et al., 2018b).

There is need for inexpensive, field-ready screening technologies to detect possible food or medicines fraud or contamination, as well as a need to decrease the cost, both direct and associated, with existing technologies (Petersen et al., 2017). Real-time polymerase chain reaction, handheld Raman, and near-infrared, all technologies with great potential to detect medicines fraud, have not been manufactured or distributed at large scale (Batson et al., 2016; Ellis et al., 2015; Fernandez et al., 2011; Hajjou et al., 2013). As a result, the process for manufacturing these technologies and distributing at scale in low- and middle-income countries has not been optimized. Because the market for such screening tools is small, the companies that make them have little incentive to invest in production. A small market also prevents companies from developing a distribution system through which equipment and consumable supplies could be imported. Lack of optimal manufacturing or an infrastructure for distribution creates a vicious cycle where small market size leads to weak incentives to invest, which keeps the market small.

Recommendation 3-5: The United States International Development Finance Corporation, the International Finance Corporation (IFC), the UK CDC Group, and the European development finance banks should provide advisory services and concessional financing to manufacturers of quality and safety screening technologies to optimize manufacturing and create stronger distribution systems in low- and middle-income countries.

Quality laboratories will always be an essential part of any product safety system. Rates of false negatives and false positives can vary for different analytic methods, and the use of rapid screening technologies should always take into account their accuracy (Lalani et al., 2017; Pan and Ba-Thein, 2018). At the same time, the promise of rapid technologies is not being realized in the parts of the world that need them most. Improvements to manufacturing and distribution systems for these technologies would foster a stronger market. The strong market would, in turn, help keep the cost of consumables and equipment competitive.

The committee also recognizes that there is still a need for more field-ready, inexpensive screening tools for food safety and medicine quality. Further investment in these tools, especially from the major scientific research funders, both private and governmental, would be welcome. Strong distribution systems and manufacturing capacity help break the cycle of small markets and weak incentives to invest; they also improve the reach of the many useful tools already developed.

More rigorous assessments of the cost-effectiveness of various screening strategies would also improve the ability of financers and manufacturers to invest in products with the best potential. Research on the cost-effectiveness of screening tools is not as well developed as for medical products, making it impossible to comment on a cost-effectiveness threshold for technologies. Furthermore, a full accounting of cost-effectiveness considers not just the technology but the strategy in which it is deployed. Therefore, a cheap tool might prove cost-*in*effective if the associated costs (e.g., staff time, transportation, consumables) are high or if it is deployed inefficiently. Research on the cost-effectiveness of various tools and strategies for their use is needed and would help in determining what screening tools are better suited to different settings.

EXPANDING THE EVIDENCE BASE FOR REGULATORY POLICY

As the previous chapter discussed, regulation of food and medicines corrects a market failure and provides a public good. The agency's ability to do this job well depends on its ability to use another public good: knowledge. But regulatory science, defined as "the science of developing new tools, standards, and approaches to assess the safety, efficacy, quality, and performance of ... regulated products," is not well-studied (Adamo et al., 2015). Developing methods for understanding risk is a part of regulatory science; it also includes tools for understanding the social and cultural aspects of regulatory decisions and the tradeoffs regulators are obliged to make (IOM, 2012b). The best practices, particularly those suited to small countries, regional consortia, or low- and middle-income countries, are not always clear. For example, the previous section discussed the use of portable screening tools to detect unsafe products in the marketplace. A recent systematic review of these tools found that while there are over 41 portable devices available for field testing of medicines, there is no research commenting on the cost-effectiveness of the various tools or where in the supply chain they should be deployed, the very questions regulators would most want answered (Vickers et al., 2018).

In preparing this report, the committee discussed advances in regulatory science, strategies for capacity building, the balance of work sharing among small or neighboring countries, optimal delegation of tasks from federal to local levels, and the ideal mix of revenue for an agency, all topics discussed further in Chapters 4 and 5. Consistently, it found that evidence to inform specific policy actions was not available. This gap can and should be corrected. Many of the regulatory agencies in the Americas for example, are less than 25 years old (Barbano, 2019). Formal, regional regulatory collaborations are even newer; the African Medicines Agency is only now forming, and the Caribbean Regulatory System Initiative started in 2014 (Cargill, 2016; IFPMA, 2018). When agencies are new, there is opportunity to start fresh with a system suitable to the context. It would be unfortunate if any of these agencies were to transfer inefficient or outdated practices, either from earlier systems or from advanced agencies, simply because no better options have been identified.

When well-resourced, established agencies face similar knowledge gaps, they have ways to collaborate with academia to advance the science they need. The FDA Centers of Excellence in Regulatory Science and Innovation is a good example of such collaboration. Since 2011, these four centers, based at universities, research priorities identified in the agency's strategic plan. They also provide a venue for regulatory staff and other experts in the field to work together on topics of shared interest (FDA, 2016, 2018a). Though occasionally criticized for being overly broad, research topics have included drug compounding, pharmacovigilance, the sharing of research data, and the use of computational modeling to understand drug metabolism (FDA, 2016, 2018a,c; Fishburn, 2014). The FDA evaluates the research produced on the basis of how well it informs the agency's decisions and, ultimately, advances public health (see Figure 3-7).

The most pressing questions in regulatory science in low- and middle-income countries are not necessarily the same as those for the FDA. Nevertheless, the model of dedicated centers or consortia to research priority questions is transferable around the world. These centers, run in collaboration with universities or consortia in low- or middle-income countries, would research product safety needs in their respective regions, as well as public policy questions related to running a regulatory agency, or strategies to improve local manufacturing or quality control. As with the centers in the United States, the dissemination of the knowledge produced would also be an important component of the work.

Recommendation 3-6: The National Institutes of Health, in collaboration with the U.S. Food and Drug Administration and the U.S. Agency for International Development, should develop a network of Global Centers of Excellence in Regulatory Science for research and capacity building to identify and address the challenges of ensuring food and drug safety in low- and middle-income countries.

In some ways, the FDA would be the more suitable agency to implement this recommendation. It has relevant experience designing extramural collaborations to advance regulatory science; it also has a meaningful stake

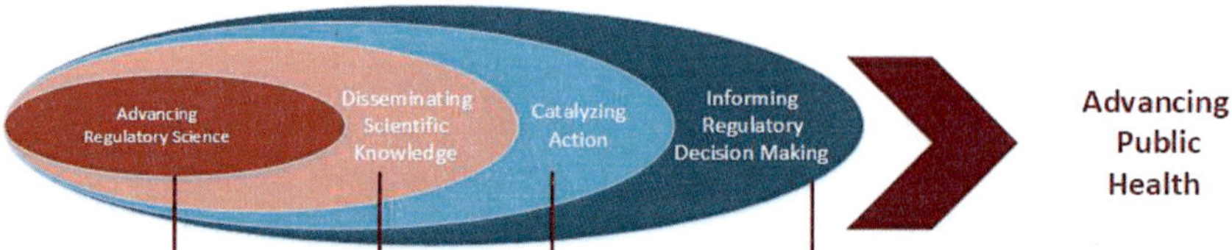

• Alignment with FDA regulatory science priority(s) • Enhancement of FDA resources, expertise, and capacity • Facilitation of strategic relationships with expert groups and stakeholders (e.g., patients, industry, professional societies, healthcare practitioners) • Building FDA preparedness for rapid response to health emergencies and new developments in emerging regulatory science through strategic social alliances	• Scientific publications and citations in literature • Presentations at conferences, meetings, or FDA Advisory Committee meetings • Incorporation into training and education curriculum • Media coverage • Data-sharing with public	• Adoption or adaptation of findings by stakeholders and use of findings in advocacy • Technology transfer to stakeholders • Subject of professional society meeting • Catalyst for future research • Improvements in consumer understanding • Adoption for use into medical practicce	Development or change in: • Reference materials and standards • Surveillance strategies • Guidelines or guidance • Regulations • Compliance and enforcement strategies • Inspection or sampling strategies • External communication strategies • Labeling • Agency Policy

FIGURE 3-7 Measures used to assess the Centers of Excellence in Regulatory Science and Innovation's research.
SOURCE: FDA, 2018b.

in the cause. The agency has existing connections with regulators in other parts of the world, both because of its involvement in international regulatory networks and through its offices in China, Europe, India, and Latin America. The National Center for Toxicological Research, for example, is a research division of the FDA that encourages collaboration with government, academic, and industry experts in the United States and abroad (FDA, 2019). The FDA also organizes an annual Global Summit on Regulatory Science to discuss the application of basic science for regulatory uses and innovative technologies affecting regulators' work (FDA, 2019). Still, a 2015 evaluation acknowledged that the agency is not generally a research funder and "has very limited funding to apply to regulatory science research and training," even domestically (FDA, 2016).

The National Institutes of Health (NIH) is a research funder; its role as such is part of its strategic reason to invest in Global Centers of Excellence in Regulatory Science. Promoting regulatory science is a way to protect the

NIH's considerable investment in global health. To put it in perspective, between 2017 and 2019 the NIH spent about $200 million a year on malaria research (separate from the almost $60 million a year on malaria vaccine), between $100 and $150 million a year on foodborne illness, and from $470 to over $550 a year on antimicrobial resistance (NIH, 2019). The agency supports about $2.5 billion a year in vaccine development, including malaria, tuberculosis, and AIDS-related vaccines (NIH, 2019). This research has generated considerable knowledge for humanity, much of it intended to improve health in low- and middle-income countries. Regulatory system failures prevent this investment from realizing its full value. If a regulatory authority cannot manage lot releases of a vaccine, for example, these products will fail to reach some intended recipients. The best knowledge about treating or preventing any illness will remain mostly academic without good-quality food and medical products on the market.

The NIH also has some experience in promoting regulatory science. Its Clinical and Translational Science Awards group has a regulatory science subgroup that, in 2014, developed a list of core thematic areas and skills for regulators; it also promoted the consortium model as well suited to a multidisciplinary field (Adamo et al., 2015). The translational science group is also active in a network of medical research institutions around the United States that collaborate on translational research, tools, and processes (NIH, 2018a). Another NIH and FDA partnership produced the Common Fund Regulatory Science Program, "a collaborative effort to accelerate the development and use of new tools, standards, and approaches" to the regulation of medical products (NIH, 2018b). There is also precedent for the NIH's involvement in Centers of Excellence in Regulatory Science. The NIH supports these centers in the United States, working with the FDA and other agencies to create more financial leverage for the programs and for other intramural projects that draw on expertise from a variety of stakeholders (FDA, 2011). The U.S. Agency for International Development (USAID) also has an interest in promoting operational research and translating that into practice in its partner countries. The agency has some experience with Centers of Excellence already; a recent program in Egypt set up partnerships between Egyptian and U.S. universities in energy, agriculture, and water (USAID, 2019d). The Center of Excellence in Agriculture, for example, is expected to "increase the quality and quantity of applied research projects that transform agricultural business" and to produce the type of research the government can use in policy making (USAID, 2019e). The investment in regulatory science would also be complementary to the agency's work in food and agriculture, as an implementer of the PEPFAR[6] program and the President's Malaria Initiative and treatment of other infectious diseases (USAID, 2019a,b,c).

---

[6] Officially, the President's Emergency Plan for AIDS Relief.

Research in low- and middle-income countries can be criticized for being "extractive" or characterized by insufficient attention to working with researchers in the host country on local priorities (Chu et al., 2014). The committee envisions that the research priorities for the proposed centers would depend on the local needs. One way to ensure the usefulness of the research produced can be adapted from the WHO's Alliance for Health Policy and Systems Research. In this model, policy makers from low- and middle-income countries serve as co-principal investigators, helping to design and conduct studies (Langlois et al., 2017). This strategy helps ensure there is demand for the research produced; it can also improve implementation and scale-up (Langlois et al., 2017). The proposed Centers of Excellence should work in a similar way, involving experts from the regulatory agencies in their target country or region to ensure the research generated targets practical questions of local priority.

It is also important to emphasize that, while the centers may have a training element, they are not training centers. This distinguishes the centers proposed from existing programs, such as the Regional Centers of Regulatory Excellence affiliated with the New Partnership for Africa's Development (AUDA-NEPAD, n.d.). The main role of these centers is training regulators, at universities and through exchange programs, as well as through practicum with industry, with operational research being a lower priority (AUDA-NEPAD, n.d.). The centers envisioned in this report, in contrast, are primarily operational research centers.

In implementing this recommendation, the agencies might draw valuable lessons on collaborative centers from the Joint Institute for Food Safety and Applied Nutrition, a partnership between the University of Maryland and the FDA to increase good-quality research on food safety and human, animal, and plant health (JIFSAN, n.d.-a). Some collaborations, such as one on spice safety in India, have required partnership with the host-country government, as well as with spice farmers and processors and Indian universities (JIFSAN, n.d.-b; Narrod et al., 2018). Local experts run the trainings and act as advocates for the work, mobilizing local funding and developing ways to monitor and evaluate the results of their work (JIFSAN, n.d.-b). Similar work with the Bangladesh Shrimp and Fish Foundation has helped ensure that information about safe aquaculture has reached as large an audience as possible (JIFSAN, n.d.-a). The common thread to both programs is the emphasis on local ownership. In both settings, the training of trainers approach helped improve reach, while tools such as demonstration farms can be used for teaching long after the program ends (Narrod et al., 2018; Spices Board India, 2015).

There are also transferable lessons to be drawn from USAID's Global Innovation Labs, especially the Partnerships for Enhanced Engagement in Research piece of these labs. Like the centers proposed, the Global

Innovation Labs support scientists in developing countries to conduct research in areas important to the USAID. These partnerships draw on investments from other U.S. government agencies, including the NIH and the USDA (USAID, 2018). For example, the program supported researchers in Tanzania and North Carolina who mapped the geographical distribution of certain viruses that affect cassava, allowing district governments in Tanzania to issue effective quarantines, thereby protecting susceptible crops (USAID, 2018).

Several places in this report highlight research gaps that affect regulators. These may be questions the proposed Centers of Excellence would take on but, to be clear, any center's research agenda would be tailored to local demand. An initial assessment of needs and scope, involving both funders in the United States and research and policy experts in low- and middle-income countries, would be part of the implementation of this recommendation.

REFERENCES

Abraham, F., and S. L. Schmukler. 2017. *Addressing the SME finance problem.* Washington, DC: The World Bank Group.

Abuka, C., R. K. Alinda, C. Minoiu, J.-L. Peydró, and A. F. Presbitero. 2019. Monetary policy and bank lending in developing countries: Loan applications, rates, and real effects. *Journal of Development Economics* 139:185–202.

Adamo, J. E., E. E. Wilhelm, and S. J. Steele. 2015. Advancing a vision for regulatory science training. *Clinical and Translational Science* 8(5):615–618.

AUDA-NEPAD (African Union Development Agency-New Partnership for Africa's Development). n.d. *Regional centres of regulatory excellence (RCORES).* https://www.nepad.org/publication/what-regional-centres-regulatory-excellence-rcores (accessed November 6, 2019).

Avant, S. 2018. *Building a one-stop system for food data.* https://agresearchmag.ars.usda.gov/2018/mar/food/#printdiv (accessed November 25, 2019).

Barbano, D. B. 2019. *ANVISA—Brazil's national health surveillance agency.* Paper read at Committee on Stronger Food and Drug Regulatory Systems Abroad, January 25, 2019, Costa Rica.

Batson, J. S., D. K. Bempong, P. H. Lukulay, N. Ranieri, R. D. Satzger, and L. Verbois. 2016. Assessment of the effectiveness of the CD3+ tool to detect counterfeit and substandard anti-malarials. *Malaria Journal* 15(1):119.

Branigan, D. 2019. *WHO benchmarking tool made "more transparent" in evaluating regulatory authorities.* https://www.healthpolicy-watch.org/who-benchmarking-tool-made-more-transparent-in-evaluating-regulatory-authorities (accessed November 11, 2019).

Caipo, M. 2019, *FAO/WHO Food Control System Assessment Tool.* Paper presented at Committee on Stronger Food and Drug Regulatory Systems Abroad, February 25, San Jose, Costa Rica.

Cargill, L. 2016. *The Caribbean regulatory system initiative.* Paper read at VIII Conference of the PANDRH, Mexico City.

CDC (U.S. Centers for Disease Control and Prevention). n.d. *Medaccess: Increasing access to crucial medical supplies in Africa and South Asia.* https://www.cdcgroup.com/en/how-we-invest/how-we-partner-with-businesses/initiatives/medaccess (accessed September 20, 2019).

Chatterjee, S. 2012. *FDA perspective on continuous manufacturing.* Paper read at IFPAC Annual Meeting, January 2012, Baltimore, MD.

Chen, C., F. Zhang, J. Barras, K. Althoefer, S. Bhunia, and S. Mandal. 2016. Authentication of medicines using nuclear quadrupole resonance spectroscopy. *IEEE/ACM Transactions on Computational Biology and Bioinformatics* 13(3):417–430.

Chu, K. M., S. Jayaraman, P. Kyamanywa, and G. Ntakiyiruta. 2014. Building research capacity in Africa: Equity and global health collaborations. *PLoS Medicine* 11(3):e1001612.

Clay, E. J., M. Geddes, and L. Natali. 2009. *Aid untying: Is it working? Thematic study on the developmental effectiveness of untied aid: Evaluation of the implementation of the Paris declaration and of the 2001 DAC recommendation on untying ODA to the LDCS.* Copenhagen, Denmark: Overseas Development Institute.

Comerford, M. 2018. How continuous processing is impacting U.S. drug manufacturing facilities. Site Selectors Guild. https://www.tradeandindustrydev.com/industry/bio-pharmaceuticals/how-continuous-processing-impacting-us-drug-manufa-13749 (accessed September 20, 2019).

Crossette, B. 2019. Unsafe food, a killer in poor nations, needs government action. PassBlue. https://www.passblue.com/2019/02/06/unsafe-food-a-killer-in-poor-nations-needs-government-action (accessed July 17, 2019).

Davidson, J. G. 2016. *The real cost of poor data integrity in pharmaceutical manufacturing.* Westbury, NY: Lachman Consultant Services, Inc. https://www.lachmanconsultants.com/wp-content/uploads/2016/05/data-integrity-whitepaper.pdf (accessed December 8, 2019).

de Ronzio, P. 2016. *Accountability dilemmas in foreign aid.* London, UK: Overseas Development Institute.

Dellepiane, N., and D. Wood. 2015. Twenty-five years of the WHO vaccines prequalification programme (1987–2012): Lessons learned and future perspectives. *Vaccine* 33(1):52–61.

Digital Campus Moodle. 2016. *Ethiopia's One WaSH National Programme.* https://moodle.digital-campus.org/mod/page/view.php?id=32972 (accessed November 22, 2019).

Elliott, K. A. 2019. *Developing a more inclusive U.S. trade policy at home and abroad.* Washington, DC: Center for Global Development.

Ellis, D. I., H. Muhamadali, S. A. Haughey, C. T. Elliott, and R. Goodacre. 2015. Point-and-shoot: Rapid quantitative detection methods for on-site food fraud analysis—Moving out of the laboratory and into the food supply chain. *Analytical Methods* 7(22):9401–9414.

EMA (European Medicines Agency). 2019. *Big data.* https://www.ema.europa.eu/en/about-us/how-we-work/big-data (accessed July 18, 2019).

Fair, R. J., and Y. Tor. 2014. Antibiotics and bacterial resistance in the 21st century. *Perspectives in Medicinal Chemistry* 6:25–64.

FAO (Food and Agricultural Organization of the United Nations). 2014. *Assessing national food control systems: Measuring effectiveness and planning for improvements.* http://www.fao.org/3/a-ml734e.pdf (accessed August 22, 2019).

FAO. 2017a. Preparing a national phytosanitary capacity development strategy. http://www.fao.org/3/i7766en/I7766EN.pdf (accessed January 16, 2020).

FAO. 2017b. *Harnessing rather than suppressing informal trade can give Africa a boost: FAO study offers policy guidance for linking half of all cross-border trade to development goals.* http://www.fao.org/news/story/en/item/888767/icode (accessed July 19, 2019).

FAO. 2019. *FAO and WHO support performance assessment of Tunisia's national food control system.* http://www.fao.org/neareast/news/view/en/c/1189851 (accessed July 18, 2019).

FAO and WHO (World Health Organization). 2019a. FAO/WHO Food Control System Assessment Tool. *Codex Alimentarius International Food Standards*, July 7, 2019.

FAO and WHO. 2019b. *Food Control System Assessment Tool: Introduction and glossary*. Food safety and quality series No. 7/1. http://www.fao.org/3/ca5334en/CA5334EN.pdf (accessed July 17, 2019).

FDA (U.S. Food and Drug Administration). 2011. *Advancing regulatory science at FDA: A strategic plan*. https://www.fda.gov/science-research/science-and-research-special-topics/advancing-regulatory-science (accessed December 8, 2019).

FDA. 2016. *Centers of Excellence in Regulatory Science and Innovation (CERSIs)—Program evaluation, a report to the FDA science board from the CERSIs program evaluation subcommittee*. https://www.fda.gov/media/96457/download (accessed October 10, 2019).

FDA. 2018a. *Centers of Excellence in Regulatory Science and Innovation (CERSIs)*. https://www.fda.gov/science-research/advancing-regulatory-science/centers-excellence-regulatory-science-and-innovation-cersis (accessed July 17, 2019).

FDA. 2018b. *CERSIs research impact metrics*. https://www.fda.gov/science-research/advancing-regulatory-science/cersi-research-impact-metrics (accessed July 17, 2019).

FDA. 2018c. *CERSIs research projects*. https://www.fda.gov/science-research/advancing-regulatory-science/cersi-research-projects (accessed July 17, 2019).

FDA. 2018d. *Mutual recognition agreement (MRA)*. https://www.fda.gov/international-programs/international-arrangements/mutual-recognition-agreement-mra (accessed May 3, 2019).

FDA. 2019. *NCTR international programs and activities*. https://www.fda.gov/about-fda/science-research-nctr/nctr-international-programs-and-activities (accessed August 21, 2019).

Fernandez, A. 2019. *Advancing food safety with technology and traceability*. https://www.foodsafetymagazine.com/enewsletter/advancing-food-safety-with-technology-and-traceability (accessed September 23, 2019).

Fernandez, F. M., D. Hostetler, K. Powell, H. Kaur, M. D. Green, D. C. Mildenhall, and P. N. Newton. 2011. Poor quality drugs: Grand challenges in high throughput detection, countrywide sampling, and forensics in developing countries. *The Analyst* 136(15):3073–3082.

Fishburn, C. S. 2014. Go west, FDA. *Science-Business eXchange* 7(22):632.

FMO (Netherlands Development Finance Company). 2016. *Investments in infrastructure manufacturing and services*. https://www.fmo.nl/l/library/download/urn:uuid:27a2c590-125c-4d3b-9eab-324d53b10d2b/20161220+ims+evaluation+report.pdf (accessed October 29, 2019).

FMO. 2018. *Agribusiness sector evaluation 2018*. https://www.fmo.nl/l/library/download/urn:uuid:2a93e6fe-6bf1-4d81-acc3-c7b7ed45a80b/sector+evaluation+report+fmo+def+version.pdf (accessed October 29, 2019).

FSA (Food Standards Agency). 2019. *Chief scientific adviser's report reveals the data standards enhancing food safety*. https://www.food.gov.uk/news-alerts/news/chief-scientific-advisers-report-reveals-the-data-standards-enhancing-food-safety (accessed July 19, 2019).

FSN (*Food Safety News*). 2019. *World Bank Group supports projects to improve African food safety*. https://www.foodsafetynews.com/2019/06/world-bank-group-supports-projects-to-improve-african-food-safety (accessed August 27, 2019).

Gascó, M., W. Feng, and J. R. Gil-Garcia. 2018. *Providing public value through data sharing: Understanding critical factors of food traceability for local farms and institutional buyers*. Paper presented at the January 2018 Hawaii International Conference on System Sciences, University of Hawaii at Manoa.

GFSI (Global Food Safety Initiative). 2018. *Global Food Safety Initiative (GFSI) announces global partnership with international finance corporation*. https://www.prnewswire.com/news-releases/global-food-safety-initiative-gfsi-announces-global-partnership-with-international-finance-corporation-675956203.html (accessed September 20, 2019).

Global Industry Analysts Inc. 2019. *Growing need to prevent foodborne illness amidst implementation of stringent foods safety regulations continues to drive growth in the food safety testong market.* https://www.strategyr.com/MarketResearch/market-report-infographic-food-safety-testing-forecasts-global-industry-analysts-inc.asp (accessed October 29, 2019).

Grace, D., K. Makita, E. Kang'ethe, B. Bonfoh, and K. Roesel. 2014. Taking food safety to informal markets. In *Food safety and informal markets: Animal products in sub-Saharan Africa*, edited by K. Roesel and D. Grace. London, UK: Routledge. Pp. 1–8.

GS1 US. 2016. *USDA branded food products database created to expand the USDA national nutrient database.* https://www.prnewswire.com/news-releases/usda-branded-food-products-database-created-to-expand-the-usda-national-nutrient-database-300330957.html (accessed September 9, 2019).

Guzman, J. 2019. *Driving investments in the regulatory agency: The case of Colombia.* http://www.nationalacademies.org/hmd/~/media/Files/Activity%20Files/Global/Stronger-Regulations/Meeting%202/Guzman_Driving%20investments%20in%20the%20regulatory%20agency_Javier%20Guzman.pdf (accessed July 19, 2019).

Hajjou, M., Y. Qin, S. Bradby, D. Bempong, and P. Lukulay. 2013. Assessment of the performance of a handheld raman device for potential use as a screening tool in evaluating medicines quality. *Journal of Pharmaceutical and Biomedical Analysis* 74:47–55.

Hale, T., and D. Held, eds. 2011. *Handbook of transnational governance: Institutions and innovations.* Cambridge, UK: Polity Press.

Henson, S., and J. Humphrey. 2010. Understanding the complexities of private standards in global agri-food chains as they impact developing countries. *Journal of Development Studies* 46(9):1628–1646.

IADB (Inter-American Development Bank). 2017. *Breve 18, based on the webinar, procurement policies for pharmaceuticals: The international experience.* https://publications.iadb.org/publications/english/document/Breve-18-Procurement-Policies-for-Pharmaceuticals-The-International-Experience.pdf (accessed December 8, 2019).

ICDRA (International Conference of Drug Regulatory Authorities). 2016. *Recommendations.* Paper read at 14th International Conference of Drug Regulatory Authorities, Singapore.

ICDRA. 2018. *Smart safety surveillance: A life-cycle approach to promoting safety of medical products.* Paper read at 18th International Conference of Drug Regulatory Authorities, Dublin.

IFC (International Finance Corporation). 2018. *Technology helps African farmers sell what they sow.* https://www.ifc.org/wps/wcm/connect/news_ext_content/ifc_external_corporate_site/news+and+events/news/impact-stories/technology-helps-african-farmers-sell-what-they-sow (accessed August 27, 2019).

IFC. n.d.-a. *Advice.* https://www.ifc.org/wps/wcm/connect/CORP_EXT_Content/IFC_External_Corporate_Site/Solutions/Products+and+Services/Advisory (accessed September 20, 2019).

IFC. n.d.-b. *SME finance.* https://www.ifc.org/wps/wcm/connect/Industry_EXT_Content/IFC_External_Corporate_Site/Financial+Institutions/Priorities/SME+Finance (accessed September 20, 2019).

IFPMA (International Federation of Pharmaceutical Manufacturers and Associations). 2018. *IFPMA welcomes set-up of new African Medicines Agency.* Geneva, Switzerland. https://www.ifpma.org/resource-centre/ifpma-welcomes-set-up-of-new-african-medicines-agency (accessed December 8, 2019).

IHME (Institute for Health Metrics and Evaluation). n.d. *Global burden of disease (GBD).* http://www.healthdata.org/gbd (accessed September 20, 2019).

ILSI (International Life Sciences Institute). n.d. *USDA global branded food products database*. http://ilsina.org/wp-content/uploads/sites/6/2019/07/USDA-Global-BFPD-1-Pager-June-2019.pdf (accessed September 9, 2019).

IOM (Institute of Medicine). 2012a. *Ensuring safe foods and medical products through stronger regulatory systems abroad*. Washington, DC: The National Academies Press.

IOM. 2012b. The importance of innovative regulatory science. In *Strengthening a workforce for innovative regulatory science in therapeutics development: Workshop summary*. Washington, DC: The National Academies Press.

IOM. 2013. *Countering the problem of falsified and substandard drugs*. Washington, DC: The National Academies Press.

IOM and NRC (National Research Council). 2010. Adopting a risk-based decision-making approach to food safety. In *Enhancing food safety: The role of the food and drug administration*. Washington, DC: The National Academies Press. P. 588.

IRPCV (Italian Regional Pharmacovigilance Center of Veneto). 2018. *The role of big data in pharmacovigilance*. https://www.pharmaco-vigilance.eu/content/role-big-data-pharmacovigilance (accessed July 18, 2019).

Jaffee, S., S. Henson, L. Unnevehr, D. Grace, and E. Cassou. 2019. *The safe food imperative: Accelerating progress in low- and middle-income countries. Agriculture and food series*. Washington, DC: World Bank.

Jahnke, R. 2018. Letter to the editor on previously published GPHF-minilab assessment. *American Journal of Tropical Medicine and Hygiene* 98(6):1880.

JIFSAN (Joint Institute for Food Safety and Applied Nutrition). n.d.-a. *Aquatic and aquacultural food safety center*. http://international.jifsan.umd.edu/aquatic-and-aquacultural-food-safety-center (accessed July 17, 2019).

JIFSAN. n.d.-b. *The SCMSBI program*. https://international.jifsan.umd.edu/scmsbi (accessed July 17, 2019).

Kaddu, G., E. D'Amore, A. Clark, and P. Nkansah. 2018. *Strengthening regulatory systems to improve medical product quality in low- and middle-income countries*. Rockville, MD: Promoting the Quality of Medicines (PQM) program. U.S. Pharmacopeial Convention.

Karim, M., and J. Buckley. 2015. *Overview of recent literature on mobilizing private investment in developing countries*. EPS-PEAKS. https://assets.publishing.service.gov.uk/media/57a0899ae5274a27b2000179/Overview_of_recent_literature_on_mobilizing_private_investment_in_developing_countries.pdf (accessed December 8, 2019).

Kelesidis, T., and M. E. Falagas. 2015. Substandard/counterfeit antimicrobial drugs. *Clinical Microbiology Reviews* 28(2):443–464.

Kenny, C. 2016. What is effective aid?: How would donors allocate it? World Bank Policy Research Working Paper 4005, September 2006.

Khadem, A. 2018. *Building regulatory capacity in countries to improve the regulation of health products*. Geneva, Switzerland: World Health Organization. https://www.who.int/medicines/technical_briefing/tbs/TBS2018_RSS_Capacity_Building_CRSgroup.pdf (accessed July 25, 2019).

Knack, S., and A. Rahman. 2007. Donor fragmentation and bureaucratic quality in aid recipients. *Journal of Development Economics* 83:176–197.

Kovacs, S., S. E. Hawes, S. N. Maley, E. Mosites, L. Wong, and A. Stergachis. 2014. Technologies for detecting falsified and substandard drugs in low and middle-income countries. *PLoS One* 9(3):e90601.

Kretser, A., D. Murphy, and P. Starke-Reed. 2017. A partnership for public health: USDA branded food products database. *Journal of Food Composition and Analysis* 64:10–12.

Lalani, M., F. E. Kitutu, S. E. Clarke, and H. Kaur. 2017. Anti-malarial medicine quality field studies and surveys: A systematic review of screening technologies used and reporting of findings. *Malaria Journal* 16(1):197.

Langlois, E., N. Nhan, A. Ghaffar, L. Reveiz, and B.-P. F. 2017. Embedding research in health policy and systems in the Americas. *Revista Panamericana de Salud Pública* 41.

Martin, D. 2017. *FDA approaches to analytical challenges posed by big data.* https://www.ema.europa.eu/en/documents/presentation/presentation-fda-approaches-analytical-challenges-posed-big-data-david-martin_en.pdf (accessed December 8, 2019).

Marvin, H. J. P., E. M. Janssen, Y. Bouzembrak, P. Hendriksen, and M. Staats. 2016. Big data in food safety: An overview. *Critical Reviews in Food Science and Nutrition* 57(11).

Massa, I. 2011. *Impact of multilateral development finance institutions on economic growth.* London, UK: Overseas Development Institute.

Mathauer, I., E. Dale, and B. Meessen. 2017. *Strategic purchasing for UHC: Key policy issues and questions, a summary from expert and practitioners' discussions.* Geneva, Switzerland: World Health Organization.

MedAccess. n.d. *What we do.* https://medaccess.org/what-we-do/#a-solution (accessed November 22, 2019).

Meeks, P. 2017. *Unravelling tied aid: Why aid must never be tied to donor country companies at the expense of women and men living in poverty.* Brussels, Belgium: Eurodad.

Narrod, C., X. Dou, and C. Wychgram. 2018. *Lessons learned from JIFSAN's collaborative training centers experience promoting country driven food safety capacity building in Bangladesh and India.* Report prepared for World Bank study on making the Case for Food Safety Investment in Developing Countries.

Nayyar, G. M., L., A. Attaran, J. P. Clark, M. J. Culzoni, F. M. Fernandez, J. E. Herrington, M. Kendall, P. N. Newton, and J. G. Breman. 2015. Responding to the pandemic of falsified medicines. *American Journal of Tropical Medicine and Hygiene* 92(6 Suppl):113–118.

Ndomondo-Sigonda, M., J. Miot, S. Naidoo, A. Dodoo, and E. Kaale. 2017. Medicines regulation in Africa: Current state and opportunities. *Society of Pharmaceutical Medicine* 31(6):383–397.

NIH (National Institutes of Health). 2018a. *About the CTSA program.* https://ncats.nih.gov/ctsa/about (accessed August 21, 2019).

NIH. 2018b. *Program snapshot.* https://commonfund.nih.gov/regulatoryscience (accessed August 21, 2019).

NIH. 2019. *Estimates of funding for various research, condition, and disease categories (RCDC).* https://report.nih.gov/categorical_spending.aspx#top (accessed July 17, 2019).

OECD (Organisation for Economic Co-operation and Development). 2003. *Glossary of statistical terms: Congressional loans.* http://www.imf.org/external/pubs/ft/eds/Eng/Guide/index.htm (accessed October 2, 2019).

OECD. 2015. *Building more effective, accountable, and inclusive institutions for all.* Element 6, Paper 1. https://www.oecd.org/dac/_POST-2015%20effective%20and%20accountable%20institutions.pdf (accessed October 29, 2019).

OECD. 2017. *2017 Report on DAC untying recommendation.* DCD/DAC(2017)6/FINAL. http://www.oecd.org/dac/financing-sustainable-development/development-finance-standards/2017-Report-DAC-Untying.pdf (accessed October 29, 2019).

OECD. 2019. *Revised DAC recommendation on untying ODA.* DCD/DAC(2018)33/FINAL. https://one.oecd.org/document/DCD/DAC(2018)33/FINAL/en/pdf (accessed October 11, 2019).

OECD. n.d.-a. *Paris declaration and ACCRA agenda for action.* https://www.oecd.org/dac/effectiveness/parisdeclarationandaccraagendaforaction.htm (accessed July 17, 2019).

OECD. n.d.-b. *Untied aid.* http://www.oecd.org/dac/financing-sustainable-development/development-finance-standards/untied-aid.htm (accessed July 25, 2019).

OIE (World Organisation for Animal Health). 2017. *PVS pathway, 10 years together to improve veterinary services.* https://www.oie.int/for-the-media/press-releases/detail/article/pvs-pathway-10-years-together-to-improve-veterinary-services (accessed November 22, 2019).

OIE. 2019. *OIE tool for the evaluation of performance of veterinary services: PVS tool seventh edition.* Paris, France: World Organisation for Animal Health.

OIE. n.d.-a. *PVS gap analysis reports.* https://www.oie.int/solidarity/pvs-gap-analysis/pvs-gap-analysis-reports (accessed November 22, 2019).

OIE. n.d.-b. *The PVS gap analysis tool.* https://www.oie.int/en/solidarity/pvs-gap-analysis/pvs-gap-analysis-tool (accessed November 22, 2019).

Omondi, G. 2019. *Twiga to boost food safety drive with sh1bn support from IFC.* https://www.businessdailyafrica.com/corporate/companies/Twiga-to-boost-food-safety-drive/4003102-5143834-25ai3dz/index.html (accessed August 27, 2019).

Osondu, O., and G. Yamey. 2019. Aid effectiveness in the sustainable development goals era comment on it's about the idea hitting the bull's eye: How aid effectiveness can catalyse the scale-up of health innovations." *International Journal of Health Policy and Management* 8(3):184–186.

Pan, H., and W. Ba-Thein. 2018. Re: "Diagnostic accuracy of global pharma health fund minilab in assessing pharmacopoeial quality of antimicrobials." *American Journal of Tropical Medicine and Hygiene* 98(6):1881.

Papadavid, P. 2017. *Financing for manufacturing: Financing conditions in sub-Saharan Africa.* Supporting Economic Transformation.

Petersen, A., N. Held, L. Heide, and the Difäm-EPN Minilab Survey Group. 2017. Surveillance for falsified and substandard medicines in Africa and Asia by local organizations using the low-cost GPHF minilab. *PLoS One* 12(9):e0184165.

Pharma Boardroom. 2017. *Interview: Javier Humberto Guzmán Cruz—director general, INVIMA, Colombia.* https://pharmaboardroom.com/interviews/interview-javier-humberto-guzman-cruz-director-general-invima-colombia (accessed July 17, 2019).

Pisa, M., and D. McCurdy. 2019. *Improving global health supply chains through traceability.* Washington, DC: Center for Global Development.

Platek, S. F., N. Ranieri, and J. Batson. 2016. Applications of the FDA's counterfeit detection device (CD3+) to the examination of suspect counterfeit pharmaceutical tablets and packaging. *Microscopy and Microanalysis* 22(S3):1072–1073.

Rägo, L. 2012. *Quality of RH medicines: Update from WHO prequalification of medicines programme and beyond.* Paper read at 13th Annual Membership Meeting of the Reproductive Health Supplies Coalition, Paris.

Rasheed, H., L. Hollein, and U. Holzgrabe. 2018. Future information technology tools for fighting substandard and falsified medicines in low- and middle-income countries. *Frontiers in Pharmacology* 9:995.

Roesel, K., D. Grace, J. Kago, F. Desissa, M. Spengler, K. Amenu, J. Appiah, K. Bomfeh, C. McCrindle, C. Mwai, and A. Heeb. 2014. Farmers, traders and retailers are risk managers. In *Food safety and informal markets*, edited by K. Roesel and D. Grace. London, UK: Routledge. Pp. 69–83.

Rönninger, S., J. Berberich, V. Davoust, P. Kitz, and A. Pfenninger. 2017. The GMP/GDP inspection landscape—Part I: Data. *Pharmaceutical Technology Europe* 29(1):6–10.

Ross, J. S. 2014. *Clinical trial data sharing.* Paper read at NPA FDA Taskforce Meeting, December 15, 2014.

Roth, L., D. Bempong, J. B. Babigumira, S. Banoo, E. Cooke, D. Jeffreys, L. Kasonde, H. G. M. Leufkens, J. C. W. Lim, M. Lumpkin, G. Mahlangu, R. W. Peeling, H. Rees, M. Ndomondo-Sigonda, A. Stergachis, M. Ward, and J. Nwokike. 2018a. Expanding global access to essential medicines: Investment priorities for sustainably strengthening medical product regulatory systems. *Global Health* 14(1):102.

Roth, L., A. Nalim, B. Turesson, and L. Krech. 2018b. Global landscape assessment of screening technologies for medicine quality assurance: Stakeholder perceptions and practices from ten countries. *Global Health* 14(1):43.

Silverman, R., J. Madan Keller, A. Glassman, and K. Chalkidou. 2019. *Tackling the triple transition in global health procurement: Promoting access to essential health products through aid eligibility changes, epidemiological transformation, and the progressive realization of universal health coverage.* Washington, DC: Center for Global Development.

Spices Board India. 2015. *Spices park—the concept plan.* http://www.indianspices.com/spices-parks/spices-park-concept-plan (accessed October 7, 2019).

Stahl, M. 2013. *The WHO prequalification of medicines programme.* Paper read at CPTR 2013 Workshop, October 1–3, 2013, Washington, DC.

Starke-Reed, P. 2017. *What's new: The USDA branded food products database.* Paper read at IUNS 21st International Congress of Nutrition, October 15–20, 2017, Buenos Aires, Argentina.

STDF (Standards and Trade Development Facility). n.d.a. *Trade spillover effects: The impact on domestic food safety.* http://www.standardsfacility.org/sites/default/files/STDF_Briefing_Note_Trade_Spillovers_En.pdf (accessed July 17, 2019).

STDF. n.d.b. *Improving interventions on food safety: FAO/WHO national food control systems assessment tool* (STDF Briefing 14). http://www.standardsfacility.org/sites/default/files/STDF_Briefing_14.pdf (accessed November 11, 2019).

Susha, I., B. Rukanova, J. R. Gil-Garcia, Y.-H. Tan, and M. G. Hernandez. 2019. *Identifying mechanisms for achieving voluntary data sharing in crosssector partnerships for public good.* Paper presented at 20th Annual International Conference on Digital Government Research, Dubai, United Arab Emirates, June 18–20, 2019.

't Hoen, E. F., H. V. Hogerzeil, J. D. Quick, and H. B. Sillo. 2014. A quiet revolution in global public health: The world health organization's prequalification of medicines programme. *Journal of Public Health Policy* 35(2):137–161.

Tatay, M., and E. Torreele. 2019. Ensuring access to life-saving medicines as countries shift from global fund support. *Bulletin of the World Health Organization* 97(5):311.

TEMPO.CO. 2018. *Indonesia stands ready to implement tighter food control system.* https://en.tempo.co/read/915143/indonesia-stands-ready-to-implement-tighter-food-control-system (accessed November 11, 2019).

The Defeat-NCD (Noncommunicable Disease) Partnership. n.d.-a. *Consultative group (CG).* https://defeat-ncd.org/consultative-group-cg (accessed September 20, 2019).

The Defeat-NCD Partnership. n.d.-b. *The defeat-NCD financing facility.* https://defeat-ncd.org/our-work/the-defeat-ncd-financing-facility (accessed September 20, 2019).

The Defeat-NCD Partnership. n.d.-c. *Vision & mission.* https://defeat-ncd.org/home/visionmission (accessed September 20, 2019).

The Global Fund. 2018. *Guide to global fund policies on procurement and supply management of health products.* Geneva, Switzerland: The Global Fund.

Tyson, J. E. 2017. *Mobilising private financing for manufacturing in sub-Saharan Africa.* London, UK: Supporting Economic Transformation.

UN (United Nations). 2017. One in 10 medicines in developing countries substandard or falsified –UN health agency. *UN News.* https://news.un.org/en/story/2017/11/637781-one-10-medicines-developing-countries-substandard-or-falsified-un-health-agency (accessed February 13, 2020).

UN. n.d. *Transforming our world: The 2030 agenda for sustainable development.* https://sustainabledevelopment.un.org/content/documents/21252030%20Agenda%20for%20Sustainable%20Development%20web.pdf (accessed October 9, 2019).

Unitaid. n.d. *Support for WHO prequalification of diagnostics and medicines.* https://unitaid.org/project/support-prequalification-diagnostics-medicines/#en (accessed July 19, 2019).

Unnevehr, L., and L. Ronchi. 2014. *Food safety standards, economic and market impacts in developing countries*. Washington, DC: The World Bank Group.

USAID (U.S. Agency for International Development). 2018. *Partnerships for enhanced engagement in research (PEER)*. https://www.usaid.gov/sites/default/files/documents/15396/Fact_Sheet_-_Final_2-16-2018_1.pdf (accessed November 25, 2019).

USAID. 2019a. *Agriculture and food security*. https://www.usaid.gov/what-we-do/agriculture-and-food-security (accessed October 2, 2019).

USAID. 2019b. *Global health*. https://www.usaid.gov/global-health (accessed October 2, 2019).

USAID. 2019c. *Malaria*. https://www.usaid.gov/global-health/health-areas/malaria (accessed October 2, 2019).

USAID. 2019d. *Partnering with American universitiees to create Centers of Excellence in Energy, Water, and Agriculture in Egypt: Fact sheet*. https://www.usaid.gov/news-information/press-releases/mar-26-2019-fact-sheet-partnering-american-universities-create-centers-excellence-energy (accessed October 2, 2019).

USAID. 2019e. *Project fact sheet: Center of Excellence for Agriculture* (accessed October 2, 2019).

Vickers, S., M. Bernier, S. Zambrzycki, F. M. Fernandez, P. N. Newton, and C. Caillet. 2018. Field detection devices for screening the quality of medicines: A systematic review. *BMJ Global Health* 3(4):e000725.

Vital Strategies. n.d. *Controlling high blood pressure will save millions of lives*. https://www.resolvetosavelives.org/hypertension (accessed September 20, 2019).

Wagner, A. K., J. D. Quick, and D. Ross-Degnan. 2014. Quality use of medicines within universal health coverage: Challenges and opportunities. *BMC Health Services Research* 14:357.

Ward, M. 2019. *WHO Global Benchmarking Tool*. Paper read at Committee on Stronger Food and Drug Regulatory Systems Abroad, January 8, Washington, DC.

WBG (The World Bank Group). 2018. *Sustainable financing for sustainable development: World Bank Group capital package proposal*. Washington, DC: The World Bank Group.

WHA (World Health Assembly). 2014. Regulatory system strengthening for medical products: Agenda item 15.6. Paper read at Sixty-seventh World Health Assembly, May 24, Geneva, Switzerland.

Whitworth, J. 2018. *Experts say consumers must demand improved food safety in Africa*. https://www.foodsafetynews.com/2018/09/experts-say-consumers-must-demand-improved-food-safety-in-africa (accessed July 25, 2019).

WHO (World Health Organization). 2012. *International regulatory harmonization*. Paper read at 15th International Conference of Drug Regulatory Authorities (ICDRA), October 23–26, Tallinn, Estonia.

WHO. 2013. *Progress report: WHO prequalification*. Geneva, Switzerland: World Health Organization.

WHO. 2015. *WHO estimates of the global burden of foodborne diseases: Foodborne disease burden epidemiology reference group 2007–2015*. Geneva, Switzerland: World Health Organization.

WHO. 2017. *A study on the public health and socioeconomic impact of substandard and falsified medical products*. Geneva, Switzerland: World Health Organization.

WHO. 2019a. *Delivering quality-assured medical products for all 2019–2023: WHO's five-year plan to help build effective and efficient regulatory systems*. Geneva, Switzerland: World Health Organization.

WHO. 2019b. *Impact assessment of WHO prequalification and systems supporting activities*. Geneva, Switzerland: World Health Organization.

WHO. 2019c. *Medicines/finished pharmaceutical products*. Geneva, Switzerland: World Health Organization.

WHO. 2019d. *A new model for regulatory system strengthening*. https://www.who.int/medicines/areas/quality_safety/regulation_legislation/rss_new-model/en (accessed August 21, 2019).

WHO. 2019e. *World health organization model list of essential medicines, 21st list*. https://apps.who.int/iris/bitstream/handle/10665/325771/WHO-MVP-EMP-IAU-2019.06-eng.pdf?ua=1 (accessed August 19, 2019).

WHO. n.d.-a. *Key facts about the WHO prequalification project*. https://www.who.int/3by5/prequal/en (accessed July 16, 2019).

WHO. n.d.-b. *Medicines/finished pharmaceutical products*. https://extranet.who.int/prequal/content/prequalified-lists/medicines (accessed February 13, 2020).

WHO. n.d.-c. *Post-prequalification procedures*. https://extranet.who.int/prequal/content/post-prequalification (accessed February 13, 2020).

WHO. n.d.-d. *Prequalification*. https://www.who.int/medicines/regulation/prequalification/en (accessed July 18, 2019).

WHO. n.d.-e. *Quality control laboratories*. https://extranet.who.int/prequal/information/quality-control-laboratories (accessed July 19, 2019).

WHO. n.d.-f. *Regulatory agencies*. https://extranet.who.int/prequal/information/regulators (accessed October 1, 2019).

WHO. n.d.-g. *WHO global benchmarking tool (GBT) for evaluation of national regulatory systems*. https://www.who.int/medicines/regulation/benchmarking_tool/en (accessed July 12, 2019).

WHO. n.d.-h. *WHO prequalification financing model—questions and answers*. https://www.who.int/medicines/news/prequal_finance_model_q-a/en (accessed July 19, 2019).

Wirtz, V. J., H. V. Hogerzeil, A. L. Gray, M. Bigdeli, C. P. de Joncheere, M. A. Ewen, M. Gyansa-Lutterodt, S. Jing, V. L. Luiza, R. M. Mbindyo, H. Möller, C. Moucheraud, B. Pécoul, L. Rägo, A. Rashidian, D. Ross-Degnan, P. N. Stephens, Y. Teerawattananon, E. F. M. 't Hoen, A. K. Wagner, P. Yadav, and M. R. Reich. 2017. Essential medicines for universal health coverage. *The Lancet* 389(10067):403–476.

4

The Role of the National Government

Regulatory quality is one of the World Bank's six features of good governance, aggregate indicators of which are tracked over time to measure the institutions in a country and the way authority is exercised (Benson Wahlén, 2018; WBG, 2018b). The World Bank's indicators of regulatory quality put an emphasis on openness and the rule making process, including its use of public consultations and formal impact assessment, and the accessibility of regulations (WBG, 2018a). Like other features of good governance, the functioning of the regulatory system is partly determined by the willingness and capacity of the government in a country to enact good policies (WBG, 2018b). The same way international action and global economic trends can influence national policy, a great deal of the regulatory agency's capacity is determined at the levels above the agency itself.

Much of the regulatory agency's effectiveness, efficiency, and independence are determined by a country's political leaders, who are ultimately responsible for creating an environment conducive to product safety. This chapter discusses steps national governments can take to create an environment conducive to product safety. This includes the legal provisions that allow the regulatory system to function. It also considers different models for organizing such systems, including strategies for sharing work among countries.

Sometimes it is difficult to distinguish the role of the national government in facilitating an effective regulatory agency from the responsibility of the agency's leadership to the same end. Cooperation with foreign regulators is a responsibility of the agency, for example, but one that can only be pursued with the support of the national political leaders. Given this overlap, key concepts related to international cooperation are introduced in this chapter and revisited in Chapter 5. The value of sharing regulatory work among countries, for example, is introduced in this chapter; the steps agencies can take to operationalize such work sharing are discussed in the next chapter.

LEGAL PROTECTION

Providing a legal framework for product safety may be the most fundamental step national political leaders can take to protect food and medical products in their country. Legal provision defining the national regulatory system is the first indictor measured in the World Health Organization (WHO) Global Benchmarking Tool (WHO, 2018a). The legal provisions define what institutions are part of the regulatory system, the ways they are involved, and their ability to enforce rules (WHO, 2018a).

Momentum changing laws depends on political will, which can wax and wane over time (Ruger, 2007). Food safety in particular is not often high priority, especially in low-income countries (Jaffee et al., 2019; WHO, 2017). In such situations, convincing government of the health and economic benefits of investing in regulatory systems can help make food laws higher priority. Development partners also have role in encouraging political will. Actions such as those recommended in the previous chapter can help persuade leaders in low- and middle-income countries that investment in regulatory systems is a priority by "demonstrate[ing] that it is one" (Bollyky and Stergachis, 2013).

Assessing the level of public health protection provided by existing laws is usually the first step to passing food or medicines laws. Even when no national food or drug law exists, there are often pieces of other laws that touch on the topic (FAO, 2003; Fefer, 2012). The 2012 edition of the reference publication *Managing the Drug Supply* observed that when there are many laws on different aspects of the regulatory process, some are probably outdated, concluding, "because concepts of pharmaceutical policy are modern, legislation more than 20 years old may not be relevant; starting over may be simpler" (Fefer, 2012). It is not clear that there is a similar consensus regarding older food laws (Grace, 2015; WHO, 2017). A 2005 Food and Agriculture Organization of the United Nations (FAO) report commented that food laws in many countries "may not have been updated or may have been constantly amended creating a maze of rules which regulators, industry, and consumers find difficult to understand" (Vapnek and Spreij, 2005). Whether a country drafts new food and drug laws or revises old ones, provisions should be made for removing previous outdated laws to minimize confusion in the market (WHO, 2017).

The drafting of administrative laws is complicated, but can be eased by using model laws as examples (Fefer, 2012; WHO, 2017). The WHO has model medicines legislation, important elements of which are shown in Box 4-1. Box 4-2 shows sections of an FAO model food law for a single agency.[1] Model laws can be used as tools in reviewing and amending existing food and drug laws (UNODC, n.d.). The points shown in Boxes 4-1 and 4-2, and the publications cited, can help guide legislators through the process of drafting laws. As their name suggests, model laws are *examples*; each country is responsible for tailoring revisions to the law to suit its own needs. For this reason, the FAO is somewhat circumspect about the usefulness of model food laws (FAO, 2019). While models are useful for countries pursuing regional harmonization programs, or for governing highly technical areas, much about food and agriculture laws depend on national history (FAO, 2019). Substantial adaptions to suit local context may be necessary.

In any case, a group of legal, health, and technical experts familiar with the subject and the local context is usually needed to write or revise laws. In cases where it is not possible to assemble such a group of experts from within a country, international organizations and donors can supply them (Fefer, 2012). Knowing how to access these supports and where to draw experts from remains a challenge, however. International meetings of regulatory authorities are a useful source for consultation (Fefer, 2012), another reason why the FAO and the WHO should convene such a meeting for food regulators, as recommended in Chapter 2.

In ensuring a legal mandate for regulatory systems, legislators should give special attention to three features that help determine an agency's ability to function: independence, financial sustainability, and authority to cooperate internationally. Governments that provide these protections to their regulatory agencies do their part to foster safe, nutritious foods and good-quality medical products in their countries.

Independence

Independence is a conceptual cornerstone of a functional regulatory system designing food and drug laws. It is also necessary for consumer confidence in the system. For the purposes of running an effective regulatory system, independence refers to a lack of political interference in scientific decision making and in the hiring and firing of technical staff. As the 2012 Institute of Medicine's report *Ensuring Safe Foods and Medical Products Through Stronger Regulatory Systems Abroad* explained, an

[1] The cited document also has model laws for multiple agency systems and integrated systems.

BOX 4-1
Elements of a Comprehensive Medicines Law

A. General provisions
  1. Title*
  2. Purposes*
  3. Territorial extent
  4. Application to other laws
  5. Definitions*

B. Control of availability and marketing
  1. Drug registration*
  2. National essential medicines list/national formulary
  3. Scheduling prescription, and dispensing authority*
  4. Labeling*
  5. Genetic labeling, manufacturing, and substitution
  6. Pharmacovigilance
  7. Information and advertising*
  8. Public education
  9. Imposition fees
  10. Price control
  11. Special products (herbal medi-cines, medicines for clinical trials, orphan drugs)

C. Control of supply mechanisms
  1. Importation of medicines*
  2. Exportation of medicines*
  3. Controls, incentives, and disincen-tives for local manufacturer
  4. Control of distribution, supply, storage, and sale*

D. Drug control administration
  1. Organization and function*
  2. Appeals against decisions of the drug control authority*

E. Powers of enforcement
  1. Prohibition of specified activities*
  2. Penalties for each offense based on magnitude and occurrence*
  3. Legal procedures for offenses*

F. Powers to make rules and regulations
  1. Who has authority*
  2. Under which circumstances*

* Exemptions for which model legislation has been developed by the World Health Organization.
SOURCES: Fefer, 2012, adapted from WHO, 1998, 1999.

BOX 4-2
A Food and Agriculture Organization Model Food Law

PART I – PRELIMINARY

1. Section
2. Title
3. Interpretation

PART II – ADMINISTRATION

4. Ministerial responsibility
5. Functions of the Ministry
6. Minister's power to limit or ban substances in food
7. Minister's power to prohibit importation or cultivation
8. Minister's emergency powers
9. Minister's powers of appointment and designation
10. Establishment of National Food Board
11. Secretariat
12. Membership of the Board
13. Functioning of the Board
14. Scientific Committee

PART III – GENERAL PROVISIONS

15. Food businesses
16. Traceability
17. Hygiene rules
18. Labeling

PART IV – INSPECTIONS

19. Objects of inspections
20. Powers of authorized officers
21. Rights and duties of owners and persons in charge of food business
22. Improvement notice
23. Food unfit for consumption

PART V – IMPORT AND EXPORT

24. Requirements for imported food
25. Inspection and sampling
26. Relabeling and reconditioning

PART VI – OFFENSES AND PENALTIES

27. Sale of unwholesome food
28. Sale of food not meeting standards
29. False or misleading labeling
30. General offenses
31. Offenses by authorized officers
32. Publishing false or misleading adver-tisement
33. Offenses by bodies corporate
34. Penalties
35. Additional penalties

PART VII – OFFENSES AND PENALTIES

36. Right of appeal
37. Good faith defense
38. Presumptions
39. General defenses
40. Defenses with regard to advertisements
41. Regulations
42. Savings and repeal

SOURCE: Vapnek and Spreij, 2005.

agency's independence relates directly to the trust consumers place in it (IOM, 2012). Independence also allows industry to function with confidence that the rules affecting their products will be applied in a predictable way (IOM, 2012).

Independence does not mean, however, that the agency works in a vacuum. Regulatory decisions have a social dimension, the interpretation of which makes it important for agencies to be accountable to national leaders. As one former U.S. Food and Drug Administration (FDA) commissioner observed, "to try to take politics out of FDA, first of all will not happen, and second, should not happen. Politics basically is good if handled properly because politics reflects the views of various people in society" (Adashi et al., 2019; Gordon, 2003). It is one thing, however, to have political appointees choose the relative priorities for an agency or make decisions regarding the manner in which work is conducted. It is something else to dismiss whole cadres of technical staff en masse for political reasons (IOM, 2012). The laws establishing regulatory agencies should protect against this kind of interference and shield technical staff from undue political influence (IOM, 2012).

Part of the value of model laws, such as those presented in Boxes 4-1 and 4-2, is in creating a template to allow the agency some authority over topics that are too technical or too complicated to legislate. Provisions for independence are valuable in those areas. For example, the regulation of complex biologic medicines and their analogous generics, called biosimilars, is one of the challenges facing regulators today, including many in low- and middle-income countries (Garcia and Araujo, 2016; Godman et al., 2018; Hodkinson and Blockman, 2018). Access to these medicines may be impeded if laws affecting the approval and substitution of biosimilars or the regulator's ability to educate prescribers are overly restrictive (Falit et al., 2015). Independent regulators should be allowed to make these assessments based on scientific evidence. Biologic markets may be in particular need of greater competition. About half of the world's 100 million diabetics do not have reliable access to insulin, for example, a problem blamed in part on lack of competition among the three companies that manufacture the vast majority of the world's insulin supply (99 percent by value, 96 percent by volume) (Gotham et al., 2018; HAI, 2015).

Beyond the legal protections for regulatory agencies, a culture of openness is an investment in the agency's success. For this reason, the Organisation for Economic Co-operation and Development's (OECD's) guidance on regulatory independence, like the World Bank's indicators of regulatory governance, gives considerable attention to transparency and public consultation (OECD, 2014b; World Bank, n.d.-a). As the World Bank guidance explains, "Where citizens know the rules that govern their society and have a role in shaping them, they are more likely to comply with those rules.

Corruption is lower and the quality of regulation is higher" (World Bank, n.d.-b). Publishing the scientific basis for rules and giving the public open and advertised opportunity to comment on these rules is part of regulatory transparency, as are the terms for vetting staff for conflicts of interest (see Box 4-3).

The independence of the regulatory agency was the topic of a recent white paper from the Aspen Institute and a companion commentary in *Health Affairs* wherein seven former FDA commissioners called for a restructuring of the agency, removing it from the U.S. Department of Health and Human Services' (HHS's) authority (Aspen Institute, 2019; Califf et al., 2019). A comment on such reorganization is not within the scope of this report, nor is there evidence that an agency's relative place in the government organization predicts its successful functioning. OECD guidance on this topic emphasizes that, while independence of the regulatory agency is difficult to measure, it goes beyond its place in a government organizational chart (OECD, 2014b). A 2016 analysis of 78 medicines regulatory agencies found no relationship between an agency's structural autonomy and regulatory quality, concluding, "both good and bad regulatory systems can have semi-autonomous" structures (Pezzola and Sweet, 2016). The authors went on to note that an agency's autonomy is not necessarily related to its funding, concluding, "in developing countries guaranteed funding is much more difficult [than structural independence] to achieve" (Pezzola and Sweet, 2016).

Financial concerns were also at the center of the former FDA commissioners' recent call for reorganization (Aspen Institute, 2019). Separating

BOX 4-3
Preventing Undue Influence in Regulatory Decisions

- Was there an empirical or analytical basis for major decisions? Is the justification publicly available?
- Does the regulator conduct regular, systematic analysis of threats and opportunities?
- Can the public and regulated entities comment on these? Are they given reasonable time to respond? Is feedback from the regulator provided in response to their comments?
- In the case of exceptional treatment to regulated entities, is this communicated to other regulated entities? If not, why not?
- Is there a recusal clause for all staff and board members involved in decisions that could be perceived as not being objective?

SOURCES: OECD, 2014a, n.d.

from the HHS would, they reasoned, reduce the intermediary steps in appropriations review, ultimately guaranteeing the agency more stable and readily available funding (Aspen Institute, 2019). The budgetary barriers the former commissioners are trying to overcome may be unique to the United States, but the larger question of sustainable financing is not. The regulatory agency's independence is partly dependent on its financing, underscoring the importance of a stable and diversified revenue stream to its effective functioning (OECD, 2016b). This funding is particularly vulnerable in low- and middle-income countries (Roth et al., 2018).

Sustainable Financing

Government leaders tend to view the regulatory agency as a necessary cost center, meaning that its staffing and work are an expense with little perceived economic or political return, at least until something goes wrong. In any case, such perception is not accurate; quality, effective regulation encourages economic growth (Jalilian et al., 2007). The nature of the relationship between the agency and the economy depends on the agency's charge and the national economy. In Mexico and Brazil, the food and drug regulatory agency oversees products that account for 10 to 25 percent (respectively) of the gross domestic product (Arriola Penalosa et al., 2017; Moscou et al., 2016). In poorer countries, where essential items such as food and medicine account for a greater share of household spending, the regulatory agency may be even more prominent in the national economy (Whitmore Schanzenbach et al., 2016).

An interest in guaranteeing the financial viability of the regulatory authority should therefore be a central government priority: The agency's functioning has implications for both health and economic growth. And, because its funding at least partially determines how the agency operates, governments should give careful attention to the financing streams they authorize. Both the WHO Global Benchmarking Tool and the FAO and the WHO Food Control System Assessment Tool evaluate the financial resources that governments provide to agencies (Caipo, 2019; WHO, 2018a). Neither assessment is overly prescriptive regarding the nature of the funding streams, implicitly recognizing that there are multiple effective means to do so. Broadly speaking, most governments have a short list of sources from which to fund regulatory agencies: taxes, fees on regulated industry, earmarks, or some combination thereof. (Income in the form of fines and penalties, though revenue for the regulatory agency, are excluded from this discussion as they are not a predictable or substantial source of revenue, and because reliance on fines can create perverse incentives.)

Budgetary Subvention

Direct budgetary subvention may be the simplest way to fund the regulatory agency. It is also the means recommended by OECD, mostly because it avoids any conflict of interest that can arise from making the regulatory agency dependent on user fees (OECD, 2014b). But subvention depends on tax collection, and tax collection is challenging in low- and middle-income countries (Glenday et al., 2019; IMF, 2011). The tax base in these countries is, by definition, constrained. Still, global prosperity is increasing. As Figure 4-1 illustrates, between 2000 and 2015 the share of the world's population living in a high-income or upper-middle-income country has gone from about a quarter to slightly more than half, while the percentage living in a low-income country has shrunk by 32 percentage points (Gill et al., 2019). In theory this means the taxable income in these countries has grown. But the tax base in low- and middle-income countries can be difficult to measure, making cost-effective tax collection difficult even as governments in these countries are under pressure to provide more public services (Gill et al., 2019).

Fair and efficient tax collection is a precursor to meeting many of the Sustainable Development Goals (UN, 2018). The International Monetary Fund has long been involved in supporting governments to collect taxes (IMF, 2011). A 2011 analysis of the Fund's experience in this area emphasized the importance of political will for making progress, and the need to communicate the value of public spending to taxpayers (IMF, 2011). The value of the regulatory agency for health and consumer protection is clear and should be relatively straightforward to communicate to the public, a topic expanded on in Chapter 5. Regardless, there are many factors influencing how governments balance competing priorities in budget allocation. Even when subvention provides agencies with reliable funding, questions regarding the sufficiency of such funding may make other funding sources attractive.

User Fees

Fees "assessed to users for goods or services provided by the federal government," called user fees, are an important source of funding for many regulatory agencies (GAO, 2015). Agencies may charge for services such as application review or inspection, or tasks, such as testing samples in a laboratory. User fees are meant to apply in circumstances where the recipient benefits "beyond what is normally available to the public" (Austin, 2019). Drug companies, for example, profit from the market access regulatory approval provides *beyond* the general benefit to society from the access to any company's products. By the same token, charging for tasks in the

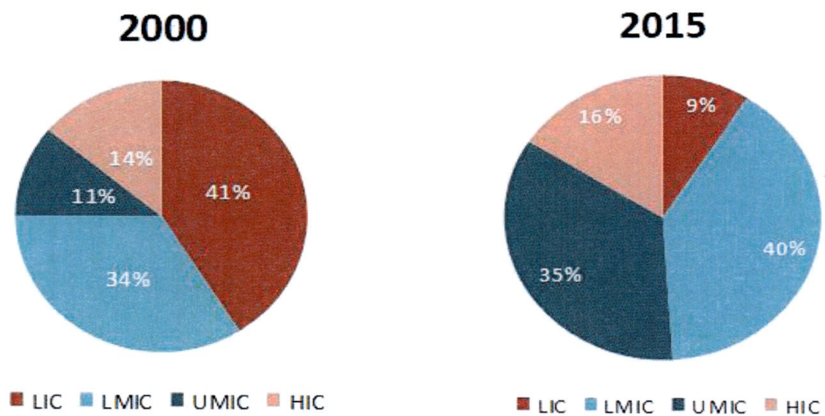

FIGURE 4-1 Distribution of world population across national income groups in 2000 and 2015.
NOTE: HIC = high-income country; LIC = low-income country; LMIC = lower-middle-income country; UMIC = upper-middle-income country.
SOURCE: Gill et al., 2019.

public interest is considered undesirable because of the risk that the charge deters use of the service. *Salmonella* testing, for example, has public benefit beyond the benefit to the requester of the test, so charging for such services may be counterproductive (MacDonald et al., 1999).

Relying on user fees to fund regulatory work is controversial, partly because it is difficult to disentangle the relative public and private benefits accrued (Austin, 2019; GAO, 2015). Even when the commercial benefit is clear and the regulatory burden easy to measure, as in the case of a drug company seeking market approval for a new molecule, user fees can alter the relationship between the regulator and industry (GAO, 1997). Almost two-thirds of the FDA's human drugs program is funded by user fees, as are about half of its total program costs (FDA, 2018). The use of fees to fund reviews has reduced the time required for market authorization of a standard new drug by about 18 months (Dabrowska and Thaul, 2018). At the same time, it has raised concerns that industry funding has influenced the agency's priorities in favor of new drug review and away from other work that does not generate revenue (Austin, 2019).

Funding the regulatory agency, especially its basic functions, from general revenues may therefore be desirable, but it is not always an option, especially in low- and lower-middle-income countries (Roth et al., 2018). A recent report on medicines regulation in Africa found that only 9 of 26 countries were funded by government (with any user fee revenue paid directly to the government treasury), but that the majority subsist on charges for market authorization and retention (Ndomondo-Sigonda et al., 2017). Drug regulatory authorities in Kenya, Malawi, Tanzania, Uganda, Zambia, and Zimbabwe receive minimal or no budgetary support from subvention (Ndomondo-Sigonda et al., 2017). A recent analysis of 95 countries' medicines regulatory agencies found that all charged some fee for registering new medicines, and that the fee charged was roughly proportional to market size (Morgan et al., 2017).

Given the pervasiveness of user fees, governments need to pay special attention to the way the system is designed, specifically to "the authority to collect and spend the revenues" (MacDonald et al., 1999). Because revenues from user fees are not always credited to the collecting agency, some may be used to fund the fee-generating program, or to offset other expenses; others are paid to the national treasury (Austin, 2019; GAO, 1997; MacDonald et al., 1999). Most agencies would have a clear preference for systems that allow them control over the fee, but legislators may dislike this, seeing an attempt to circumvent their funding authority (Austin, 2019).

Furthermore, for user fees to be acceptable to industry, charges must be a justifiable, accurate reflection of the cost of the service (GAO, 1997; MacDonald et al., 1999). Matching the incremental cost of the activity to the fee can be challenging, adjusting the fee to reflect the public benefit of the service even harder (Austin, 2019). Fees may be inaccurate if inflation increases the cost of the service, or if a new technology allows it to be done more cheaply (MacDonald et al., 1999). Underestimates on the fee schedule, even slight ones, can accumulate as an activity expands, gradually pushing an agency into deficit (MacDonald et al., 1999). It is therefore preferable that the legislature review the fee schedule every few years, as adjustments may be necessary.

Dependence on user fees can also make the agency vulnerable to market shifts. Demand for the fee-generating service may dry up, making a financial safety net in the form of government appropriations even more important (Austin, 2019; GAO, 1997). When budgetary subvention cannot provide that safety net, earmarks may be a viable stopgap.

Earmarked Revenues

In this discussion, earmarking refers to the flagging of a tax or other revenue for a specific purpose (Cashin et al., 2017; Porter and Walsh, 2006). Earmarked revenues sometimes fund programs that relate to the revenue source (e.g., using a tobacco tax to fund smoking cessation), but they may be unrelated (Porter and Walsh, 2006). Countries can also earmark a percentage of expenditures, mandating what share of the budget should be spent on health, for example. These expenditure earmarks are usually used to enforce government priorities (Cashin et al., 2017).

Earmarked taxes are a common revenue stream in low- and middle-income countries (Boakye, 2016). In places where the tax collection system is not developed, taxes on tobacco, alcohol, or unhealthy foods are seen as an effective way to fund the government's health spending (Creese, 2011).

A 2017 analysis of the use of earmarks for health emphasized that most of the arguments for and against earmarking are theoretical because, "despite vast country experience with the policy instrument—at least 80 countries earmark for health—little empirical evidence has been introduced into the debate" (Cashin et al., 2017). For these reasons, it is still not clear what circumstances are best suited to earmarking. Earmarks may work well, however, when the link between a country's stated priorities and its budget are weak because the earmark protects some revenue from competing interests (Cashin et al., 2017). Earmarks may, therefore, be a good funding option for regulatory agencies, as food and drug safety is usually a nominal priority for governments, but one that does not always translate into the budget making process.

Matching resources to priorities is a fundamental challenge of budgeting. There are administrative and economic tradeoffs to all funding options discussed in this chapter. The executive and legislative branches of government need therefore to revisit the regulatory agency's funding at regular intervals, to ensure both its sufficiency and that it is managed with efficiency and openness. Ideally, the funding for the regulatory agency should be arranged for multiple years at a time to encourage stability and prevent sudden cuts (OECD, 2014b), though in practice, almost 90 percent of regulatory agencies have single-year budgets (OECD, 2014b).

The balance of revenues that any government should use to fund its regulatory agency depends, however, on local context. Even though all countries struggle with the tradeoffs, and many with the same budgetary constraints, there is surprisingly little evidence as to what contexts are best suited to different financing strategies (Cashin et al., 2017; Ndomondo-Sigonda et al., 2017). This would be an important area for the Centers of Excellence in Regulatory Science to research. The optimal percentage of revenue regulatory agencies should draw from user fees or the conditions conducive to reliance on earmarks are the types of questions the centers might consider. Table 4-1 lists some advantages and disadvantages of various funding sources and might be a starting point for the Centers of Excellence in their research.

International Cooperation

It is important for national laws to guarantee sustainable funding to regulatory agencies because all agencies, even those with considerable resources, are facing the limits of their resources. Work sharing with foreign regulatory agencies allows countries to make more efficient use of their staff and funding. (Box 4-4 explains some important terms relevant to regulatory cooperation.) The World Health Assembly's 2014 resolution on strengthening regulatory systems encouraged member states "to engage in global, regional, and sub-regional networks of national regulatory authorities as appropriate, recognizing the importance of collaboration to pool regulatory capacities" (WHO, 2014). Like sustainable financing, a mandate for international cooperation is so central to the work of modern regulatory agencies that the WHO and the FAO benchmarking tools both assess it in their benchmarking evaluations (Caipo, 2019; WHO, 2018a). For this reason, governments should support their regulatory agencies to participate in international regulatory cooperation and harmonization programs. The drafting or revision of a country's food and drug laws is an important time to ensure these protections are in place.

When done well, regulatory harmonization serves the goal of making markets for food and medical products safer and more competitive (Pombo et al., 2016). If regulators can expand their information base through secure electronic databases, for example, the chances of an unsafe product permeating multiple markets is reduced (Allchurch et al., 2016). There are also obvious benefits to efficiency. Through sharing inspection resources,

TABLE 4-1
Pros and Cons of Different Financing Streams

	Pros	Cons
Budgetary Subvention	• Using public funds to pay for public goods • No weighting of the agency's attention in favor of revenue-earning activities	• Uncertainty in budget cycles • Process for budget approval can be lengthy • Competing demands on limited tax base
User Fees	• Direct link between payment and beneficiary • Creates fiscal space when government has competing priorities for spending tax revenue • Can improve efficiency (e.g., user fees fund more staff to review approvals, thereby decreasing review times) • Relatively predictable • Increases awareness of the cost of a service	• An incentive to emphasize activities that generate funds over other responsibilities (e.g., application review over market surveillance) • Complicates financial oversight from the legislators • Fees can be sensitive to market fluctuations • Minimum revenue needs might not be met • Risks creating a customer–client relationship between industry and regulator • Can decrease the feeling of shared responsibility for public service
Earmarked Taxes	• Safeguards funding by ring-fencing it from competing interests • Linking tax or revenue stream closely to beneficiaries may increase efficiency and soften public resistance to taxation • Increases awareness of the cost of a service	• Not easily revised or revisited; can lead to inappropriate allocation of resources • Can lead to distortions in the overall economy (e.g., if an earmarked tax is enough to dissuade people from buying the taxed product) • Funding sensitive to market fluctuations • Can limit coordination across sectors, encouraging fragmentation in budget • Can decrease the feeling of shared responsibility for public service

SOURCES: Austin, 2019; Cashin et al., 2017; GAO, 2015.

BOX 4-4
Key Definitions

Convergence: A process whereby the regulatory requirements across countries or regions become more similar over time as a result of the gradual adoption of internationally recognized technical guidance documents, standards, and scientific principles; common or similar practices and procedures; or adoption of regulatory mechanisms that might be specific to a local legal context but that align with shared principles to achieve a common public health goal. It does not necessarily represent the harmonization of laws and regulations, which is not a prerequisite for allowing the alignment of technical requirements and greater regulatory cooperation.

Harmonization: The process by which technical guidelines are developed to be uniform across participating authorities.

Reliance: The act whereby the regulatory authority in one jurisdiction may take into account and give significant weight to that is, totally or partially rely upon evaluations performed by another regulatory authority or trusted institution in reaching its own decision. The relying authority remains responsible and accountable for decisions taken, even when it relies on the decisions and information of others.

SOURCES: FDA, 2019; WHO, 2018b.

for example, regulators can substantially improve their reach. Another important benefit for heads of government to realize is that participation in regional regulatory programs strengthens national capacity (Kaddu et al., 2018). For example, the U.S. Agency for International Development and U.S. Pharmacopeia Promoting the Quality of Medicines program support joint dossier review for the East African Community (Kaddu et al., 2018). These joint reviews have clear benefits to manufacturers seeking a more streamlined process for market entry, and they advance the goal of regulatory convergence (Kaddu et al., 2018). They also involve participants from the various regulatory agencies in the region, who return to their home offices with stronger technical skills and professional relationships with colleagues abroad.

The presence of trade secret information in inspection reports can be a barrier to information sharing. There are strategies to address this barrier, however. Confidentiality agreements among agencies can enable information sharing. In 2017, for example, confidentiality agreements between the European Medicines Agency (EMA) and the FDA allowed the agencies to share inspection reports from medicines manufacturers in their respective jurisdictions and beyond, including manufacturing centers like India and China (FDAMap, 2017). Such agreements can be useful, though there are legally simpler tools, such as unilateral reliance, discussed later in this chapter, that may work better for less advanced agencies.

Low- and middle-income countries are increasingly working toward regional harmonization. Because of the economic implications for trade, regional economic communities have been leaders in harmonization, these include the East African Community, the Economic Community of West African States, the Association of Southeast Asian Nations (ASEAN), and the Asia-Pacific Economic Cooperation (Kamwanja et al., 2011; Pombo et al., 2016).

Regulatory cooperation programs are so common that even understanding the scope and goals of various and sometimes overlapping programs can be challenging. To complicate the matter, these efforts are often not well documented, especially the ones involving most low- and middle-income countries (Roth et al., 2018). Some lessons can be garnered, however, from analysis of some long-standing regulatory cooperatives in Europe and Latin America.

Examples of Regional Cooperation

The EMA, a regulatory network for European Union countries, has existed since 1995, but the legal framework supporting its work was put into place about 30 years earlier (Allchurch et al., 2016). Market authorization was the impetus for collaboration, driven by the European Community's common market (Allchurch et al., 2016). Today, EMA members rely on each other's inspection reports, clinical trials, and market surveillance data, and have pooled resources to develop electronic systems for data sharing (Allchurch et al., 2016). Fully harmonized drug laws are still a goal for EMA members, a reminder that significant meaningful cooperation is possible even without perfect equivalence among systems (Allchurch et al., 2016).

Regional regulatory harmonization and work-sharing programs in Latin American and Southeast Asia have a roughly 20-year history (Pombo et al., 2016; Teo, 2016). The Pan American Network for Drug Regulatory Harmonization and the ASEAN Pharmaceutical Product Working Groups have both made good progress producing harmonized technical guidelines for their members (Pombo et al., 2016; Teo, 2016). Both programs have also identified similar barriers to implementing these guidelines, including lack of resources and capacity (Pombo et al., 2016; Teo, 2016). If the national regulatory agency does not have enough staff, or staff with suitable training, even relatively simple guidelines can be aspirational. Other times, agencies lack the resources to follow technical guidelines. For example, guidelines on regulatory action against falsified and substandard medicines may reference detection technologies that not all agencies have (Pombo et al., 2016). Full implementation of technical guidance can also be challenging, especially when the regional guidance is intended for countries at widely different maturity levels (Pombo et al., 2016; Teo, 2016).

Donor support for harmonization, including that recommended in the previous chapter, tends to focus on removing technical barriers. Providing a secure, electronic platform for information sharing, for example, is necessary for harmonization and something donors can provide (Allchurch et al., 2016; Luigetti et al., 2016). The non-technical barriers to harmonization are more the purview of national governments. Lack of political will or trust among countries, for example, is an important non-technical barrier, and one that takes time to overcome (Luigetti et al., 2016; Rägo, 2013). There may also be legal barriers preventing regulatory authorities from participating in harmonization, if there is no legal guarantee for confidentiality, for example (Luigetti et al., 2016).

Some forms of regulatory cooperation take longer to establish then others, though none will get far without leadership from the national government. Much of the responsibility for empowering regulators to collaborate with other countries and international organizations lies with the national government. Given the increasingly global nature of food and drug markets, regulatory cooperation is crucial, especially for regulators in small or less developed countries. If done properly, regulatory processes can be harmonized across whole groups of countries, making it easier to ensure compliance with requirements, and also controlling the regulatory burden on industry.

The safety of food and medical products is one of a range of public health matters that transcend national boundaries and have political, social, and economic dimensions. The term "global health diplomacy" is used to describe such matters and the negotiations at many levels that influence health policy (Kickbusch et al., 2007). Global health diplomacy serves the goals of both protecting health and building relationships among countries (Brown et al., 2018). Attention to these relationships is an investment in solving problems that require action at both national and international levels (WHO EMRO, n.d.). Supporting its regulatory agencies is part of government's responsibility to its citizens. Political leaders can take a meaningful step to meeting that responsibility through attention to the laws that protect the regulatory agency.

Recommendation 4-1: National governments should guarantee in legislation that national regulatory agencies be independent and financially viable, with statutes that encourage cooperation with other agencies and require a scientific basis for decision making.

TABLE 4-2
Structure and Funding of a Sample of Regulatory Agencies

Country (Regulatory Agency)	Structure	Funding Source(s)	Comments
Argentina (Administración Nacional de Medicamentos Alimentos y Tecnología)	Autonomous	Subvention	Administratively and financially independent but user fees go to central funding; decision making is independent
Australia (Therapeutic Goods Administration)	Autonomous	User fees	
Ethiopia (Food and Medicine and Health Care Administration and Control Authority)	Semi-autonomous	Subvention User fees	Under Department of Health but reports to parliament
Ghana (Food and Drugs Authority)	Operationally autonomous (not financially)	Subvention User fees	Does not sit under the Ministry of Health; independent agency that reports to the minister
India (Drug Controller General of India, Drug Control Authority)	Semi-autonomous, under Ministry of Health	Subvention	Minimal user fees, which are unsustainable and provided to the ministry
Indonesia (Badan Pengawas Obat dan Makanan)	Ministry-level institution	Subvention	Minimal user fees; head of Badan Pengawas Obat dan Makanan is a minister-level position, reports to president
Lao People's Democratic Republic (Food and Drug Department)	Not autonomous, under Ministry of Health	Subvention Donors	

Netherlands (Medicines Evaluation Board)	Autonomous	User fees	Regulatory decisions are independent of ministry
Pakistan (Drug Regulatory Authority Pakistan)	Autonomous	Subvention User fees	Under Ministry of Health but independent in its decision making; minimal government funding (~2 percent)
Papua New Guinea (Pharmaceutical Service Standards Branch)	Not autonomous, under Department of Health	Subvention	Fees are returned to treasury
Singapore (Health Sciences Authority[a])	Autonomous, under Ministry of Health	Subvention User fees	Statutory board under Ministry of Health, autonomy in decision making
South Africa (South African Health Products Regulatory Authority)	Autonomous, under the Department of Health	Subvention User fees	Independent public entity that retains revenue generated, employs its own staff, and is accountable to parliament
United States of America (U.S. Food and Drug Administration [FDA])	Autonomous, under Department of Health and Human Services	Subvention User fees	Fee proportions vary by centers; decisions made almost exclusively by civil servants in the FDA (delegated decision making by law and regulation)
Zimbabwe (Medicines Control Authority of Zimbabwe)	Autonomous, not under Ministry of Health	User fees	Not under Ministry of Health, but minister is responsible for actions

[a] Health Products Regulation Group.

SOURCE: Roth et al., 2018.

In evaluating the support governments provide to their regulatory agencies, it easy to become overly focused on institutional form, if the agency operates as an autonomous or semi-autonomous division of the ministry of health, for example, or as a separate entity. There are multiple effective structures regulatory agencies can take (see Table 4-2); the best match for a particular country depends mostly on national history and context. Attention to the agencies' authority, accountability, capacity to monitor the market and enforce rules, and ability to protect public health should be the priority for legislators designing or updating a regulatory authority.

OECD guidance on regulatory policy gives some attention to the role of core policies—strategic statements from the government defining the underlying principles and governing of the regulatory agency (OECD, 2016a). The guidance emphasizes the role of the executive branch in providing

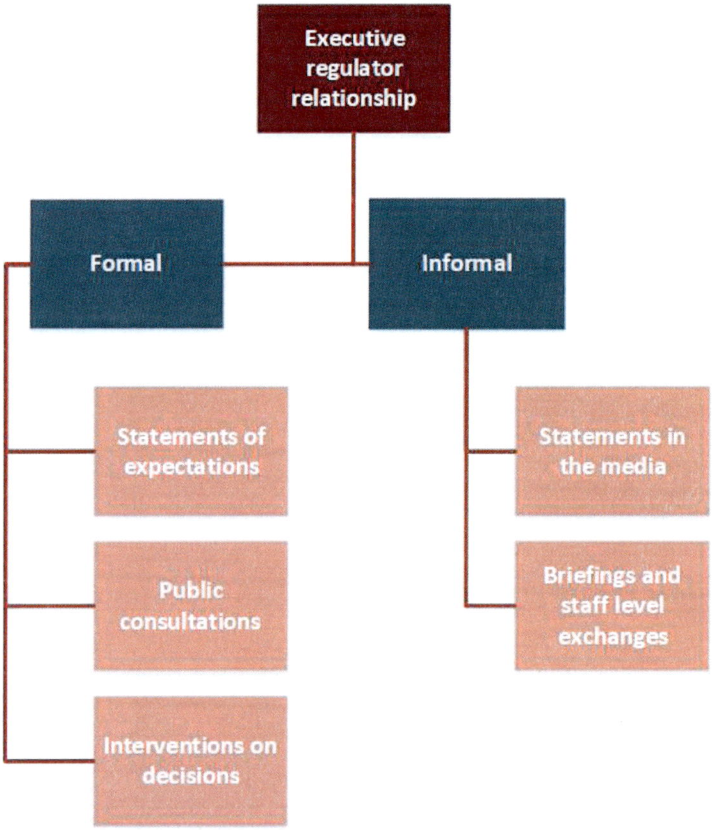

FIGURE 4-2 Interactions between regulators and the executive level of government.
SOURCE: OECD, 2016b.

clarity regarding the role and responsibilities of the regulatory agency, and in setting up a system protected from undue political interference (OECD, 2014b). Beyond the setting of expectations, the relationship between the president or parliament of a country and its regulatory agency includes various formal and informal interactions, shown in Figure 4-2 (OECD, 2016b).

OECD guidance also encourages countries to provide clear authority for coordination among regulators (OECD, 2016a). This includes coordination between the national regulatory agency and its counterparts at sub-national and local levels, as well as coordination with its counterpart agencies abroad (OECD, 2016a). The ability of regulators to work effectively across jurisdictions is central to the functioning of a modern regulatory agency.

Food and medical product regulatory decisions are made at the local, national, regional, and global levels. Some jobs, the inspection of restaurants and pharmacies, for example, must be a local responsibility, while WHO prequalification and Codex standards for international food trade are necessarily global. In determining which jobs to assign to local authorities and which ones are candidates for international collaborative action, it is important to consider possible economies of scale. Work that depends on specialized information and skills is more suitable to regional or global cooperative arrangements. For example, a local health department has an obvious responsibility for food safety in its jurisdiction, the ideas of sharing such responsibility with foreign authorities is not appropriate. Not all distinctions are so clear, and some degree of overlap, particularly between national and shared regional or global responsibilities, is inevitable (OECD, 2014b). Both ASEAN and Pan American Network for Drug Regulatory Harmonization regulators have reported problems balancing subtly competing technical guidelines from their regional regulatory collaborative and

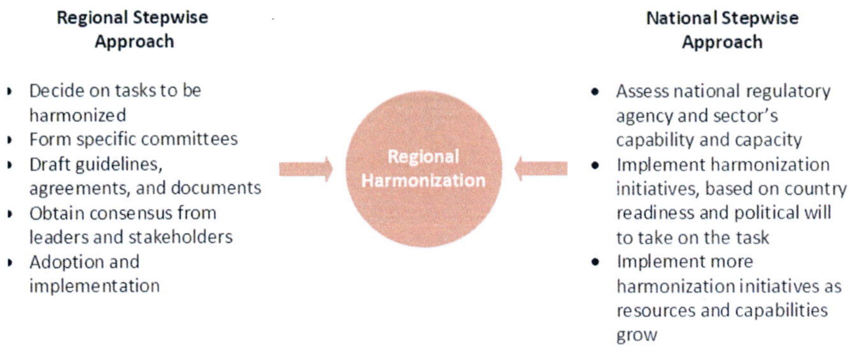

FIGURE 4-3 Stepwise approach to harmonization.
SOURCE: Teo, 2016.

global organizations such as the International Conference on Harmonization (Pombo et al., 2016; Teo, 2016). National laws can help clarify these gray areas, giving guidance on how to resolve possible conflicts (OECD, 2014b). Figure 4-3 shows steps that both national and regional authorities can take to ease the process of regulatory harmonization.

REFERENCES

Adashi, E. Y., R. S. Rajan, and I. G. Cohen. 2019. When science and politics collide: Enhancing the FDA. *Science* 364(6441):628–631.

Allchurch, M. H., D. B. Barbano, M. H. Pinheiro, and J. Lazdin-Helds. 2016. Fifty years of the European Medicines regulatory network: Reflections for strengthening intra-regional cooperation in the region of the Americas. *Revista Panamericana de Salud Pública* 39(5):288–293.

Arriola Penalosa, M. A., R. Cavazos Cepeda, M. Alanis Garza, and M. M. Lumpkin. 2017. Optimized medical product regulation in Mexico: A win-win for public and economic health. *Therapeutic Innovation and Regulatory Science* 51(6):744–750.

Aspen Institute. 2019. *Former commissioners call for the FDA to be made into an independent federal agency.* https://www.aspeninstitute.org/news/press-release/independent-fda (accessed August 9, 2019).

Austin, A. D. 2019. *Economics of federal user fees.* Washington, DC: Congressional Research Center.

Benson Wahlén, C. 2018. *World Bank updates governance indicators data set.* https://sdg.iisd.org/news/world-bank-updates-governance-indicators (accessed July 25, 2019).

Boakye, S. 2016. Revenue earmarking in Ghana: Management and performance issues. Occasional Paper Series (Institute for Fiscal Studies, Accra, Ghana).

Bollyky, T. J., and A. Stergachis. 2013. *A report of the safety and surveillance working group.* Bill & Melinda Gates Foundation. http://apps.who.int/medicinedocs/en/m/abstract/Js21347en (accessed December 8, 2019).

Brown, M. D., J. N. Bergmann, T. E. Novotny, and T. K. Mackey. 2018. Applied global health diplomacy: Profile of health diplomats accredited to the United States and foreign governments. *Global Health* 14(1):2.

Caipo, M. 2019. *FAO/WHO Food Control System Assessment Tool.* Paper presented at Committee on Stronger Food and Drug Regulatory Systems Abroad, February 25, San Jose, Costa Rica.

Califf, R. M., M. Hamburg, J. E. Henney, D. A. Kessler, M. McClellan, A. C. von Eschenbach, and F. Young. 2019. Seven former FDA commissioners: The FDA should be an independent federal agency. *Health Affairs* 38(1):84–86.

Cashin, C., S. Sparkes, and D. Bloom. 2017. Earmarking for health: From theory to practice. In WHO/HIS/HGF/HFWorkingPaper/17.5. https://www.who.int/health_financing/documents/earmarking-for-health/en (accessed February 13, 2020).

Creese, A. 2011. *WHO/HAI project on medicine prices and availability.* Geneva, Switzerland, and Amsterdam, Netherlands: WHO and HAI.

Dabrowska, A., and S. Thaul. 2018. *Prescription Drug User Fee Act (PDUFA): 2017 reauthorization as PDUFA VI.*

Falit, B. P., S. C. Singh, and T. A. Brennan. 2015. Biosimilar competition in the United States: Statutory incentives, payers, and pharmacy benefit managers. *Health Affairs (Millwood)* 34(2):294–301.

FAO (Food and Agricultural Organization of the United Nations). 2003. *Annex 6. Guidelines for developing a national food law.* www.fao.org/3/a-y8705e.pdf (accessed July 27, 2019).

FAO. 2019. *Development law—Issue #1 of 2019.* http://www.fao.org/legal/development-law/magazine-1-2019/ir/#second (accessed August 8, 2019).

FDA (U.S. Food and Drug Administration). 2018. *Fact sheet: FDA at a glance.* https://www.fda.gov/about-fda/fda-basics/fact-sheet-fda-glance (accessed April 29, 2019).

FDA. 2019. *Regulatory harmonization and convergence.* https://www.fda.gov/vaccines-blood-biologics/international-activities/regulatory-harmonization-and-convergence (accessed November 13, 2019).

FDAMap. 2017. *The practical implications of FDA and EMA sharing confidential GMP information.* https://www.fdamap.com/the-practical-implications-of-fda-and-ema-sharing-confidential-gmp-information.html (accessed September 30, 2019).

Fefer, E. 2012. Pharmaceutical legislation and regulation. In *MDS-3: Managing Access to Medicines and Health Technologies.* Arlington, VA: Management Sciences for Health.

GAO (U.S. Government Accountability Office). 1997. *Federal user fees: Budgetary treatment, status, and emerging management issues.* Washington, DC: U.S. Government Accountability Office.

GAO. 2015. *Federal user fees: Key considerations for designing and implementing regulatory fees.* Washington, DC: U.S. Government Accountability Office.

Garcia, R., and D. V. Araujo. 2016. The regulation of biosimilars in Latin America. *Current Rheumatology Reports* 18(3):16.

Gill, I., I. Bharali, and G. Glenday. 2019. *Domestic revenue mobilization: Estimating the gaps between ability and effort* (April 2019). http://centerforpolicyimpact.org/wp-content/uploads/sites/18/2019/04/CPIGH-Policy-brief_Domestic-Revenue-Mobilization__April-2019_FINAL.pdf (accessed August 5, 2019).

Glenday, G., I. Bharali, and Z. Wang. 2019. *Enhancing domestic revenues: Constraints and opportunities—a cross country comparative study of tax capacity, effort and gaps.* Durham, NC: The Center for Policy Impact in Global Health and Duke University Center for International Development.

Godman, B., A. Bucsics, P. Vella Bonanno, W. Oortwijn, C. C. Rothe, A. Ferrario, S. Bosselli, A. Hill, A. P. Martin, S. Simoens, A. Kurdi, M. Gad, J. Gulbinovic, A. Timoney, T. Bochenek, A. Salem, I. Hoxha, R. Sauermann, A. Massele, A. A. Guerra, Jr., G. Petrova, Z. Mitkova, G. Achniotou, O. Laius, C. Sermet, G. Selke, V. Kourafalos, J. Yfantopoulos, E. Magnusson, R. Joppi, M. Oluka, H. Y. Kwon, A. Jakupi, F. Kalemeera, J. O. Fadare, O. Melien, M. Pomorski, M. Wladysiuk, V. Markovic-Pekovic, I. Mardare, D. Meshkov, T. Novakovic, J. Furst, D. Tomek, C. Zara, E. Diogene, J. C. Meyer, R. Malmstrom, B. Wettermark, Z. Matsebula, S. Campbell, and A. Haycox. 2018. Barriers for access to new medicines: Searching for the balance between rising costs and limited budgets. *Frontiers in Public Health* 6:328.

Gordon, A. 2003. *The delicate dance of immersion and insulation: The politicization of the FDA commissioner.* Cambridge, MA: Harvard University.

Gotham, D., M. J. Barber, and A. Hill. 2018. Production costs and potential prices for biosimilars of human insulin and insulin analogues. *BMJ Global Health* 3(5):e000850.

Grace, D. 2015. Food safety in low and middle income countries. *International Journal of Environmental Research and Public Health* 12(9):10490–10507.

HAI (Health Action International). 2015. *Inequities and inefficiencies in the global insulin market. Fact Sheet 1.* Amsterdam, Netherlands: HAI.

Hodkinson, B., and M. Blockman. 2018. Strategies and ethics to ensure equitable access to biological medicines in the treatment of autoimmune inflammatory diseases. *Current Allergy & Clinical Immunology* 31(4).

IMF (International Monetary Fund). 2011. *Revenue mobilization in developing countries.* Washington, DC: International Monetary Fund Fiscal Affairs Department.

IOM (Institute of Medicine). 2012. *Ensuring safe foods and medical products through stronger regulatory systems abroad.* Washington, DC: The National Academies Press.

Jaffee, S., S. Henson, L. Unnevehr, D. Grace, and E. Cassou. 2019. *The safe food imperative: Accelerating progress in low- and middle-income countries.* Agriculture and food series. Washington, DC: World Bank.

Jalilian, H., C. Kirkpatrick, and D. Parker. 2007. The impact of regulation on economic growth in developing countries: A cross-country analysis. *World Development* 35(1):87–103.

Kaddu, G., E. D'Amore, A. Clark, and P. Nkansah. 2018. *Strengthening regulatory systems to improve medical product quality in low- and middle-income countries.* Rockville, MD: Promoting the Quality of Medicines (PQM) program. U.S. Pharmacopeial Convention.

Kamwanja, L. A., J. Saka, A. Awotedu, I. Fute, and M. Ndomondo-Sigonda. 2011. *Situation analysis study on medicines registration harmonisation in Africa—Final report for the economic community of West African states (ECOWAS).* Midrand, South Africa: NEPAD.

Kickbusch, I., G. Silberschmidt, and P. Buss. 2007. Global health diplomacy: The need for new perspectives, strategic approaches and skills in global health. *Bulletin of the World Health Organizaton* 85(3):230–232.

Luigetti, R., P. Bachmann, E. Cooke, and T. Salmonson. 2016. Collaboration, not competition: Developing new reliance models—regulatory collaboration. Exchange of assessment reports (ARS) with regulators outside the European Union (EU). *WHO Drug Information* 30(4):9.

MacDonald, J., F. Kuchler, J. Buzby, F. Lee, and L. Aldrich. 1999. User fees in federal agencies. In *User-fee financing of USDA meat and poultry inspection.* Washington, DC: U.S. Department of Agriculture.

Morgan, S. G., B. Yau, and M. M. Lumpkin. 2017. The cost of entry: An analysis of pharmaceutical registration fees in low-, middle-, and high-income countries. *PLoS One* 12(8):e0182742.

Moscou, K., J. C. Kohler, and A. MaGahan. 2016. Governance and pharmacovigilance in Brazil: A scoping review. *Journal of Pharmaceutical Policy and Practice* 9:3.

Ndomondo-Sigonda, M., J. Miot, S. Naidoo, A. Dodoo, and E. Kaale. 2017. Medicines regulation in Africa: Current state and opportunities. *Pharmaceutical Medicine* 31(6):383–397.

OECD (Organisation for Economic Co-operation and Development). 2014a. Being an independent regulator. In *The governance of regulators.* https://www.oecd-ilibrary.org/content/publication/9789264209015-en (accessed August 9, 2019).

OECD. 2014b. *The governance of regulators, OECD best practice principles for regulatory policy*: Paris, France: OECD Publishing.

OECD. 2016a. Governance of regulators' practices: Accountability, transparency and co-ordination. Paris, France: OECD Publishing. https://www.oecd-ilibrary.org/governance/governance-of-regulators-practices_9789264255388-en (accessed August 9, 2019).

OECD. 2016b. How does independence work in practice?: Key trends and evidence. In *Being an independent regulator*. Paris, France: OECD Publishing.

OECD. n.d. *Overview of methodologies.* https://www.oecd.org/site/schoolingfortomorrowknowledgebase/futuresthinking/overviewofmethodologies.htm (accessed October 3, 2019).

Pezzola, A., and C. M. Sweet. 2016. Global pharmaceutical regulation: The challenge of integration for developing states. *Global Health* 12(1):85.

Pombo, M. L., A. Porras, P. C. Saidon, and S. M. Cascio. 2016. Regulatory convergence and harmonization: Barriers to effective use and adoption of common standards. *Revista Panamericana de Salud Pública* 39(5):217–225.

Porter, R., and S. Walsh. 2006. *Earmarks in the federal budget process.* Cambridge, MA: Harvard Law School.

Rägo, L. 2013. *Reflections on the experiences of the World Health Organization.* Washington, DC: National Academies of Sciences, Engineering, and Medicine. http://www.nationalacademies.org/hmd/Activities/Research/DrugForum/2013-FEB-13/Day 2/Session 4/28-Rago-Video.aspx (accessed September 12, 2019).

Roth, L., D. Bempong, J. B. Babigumira, S. Banoo, E. Cooke, D. Jeffreys, L. Kasonde, H. G. M. Leufkens, J. C. W. Lim, M. Lumpkin, G. Mahlangu, R. W. Peeling, H. Rees, M. Ndomondo-Sigonda, A. Stergachis, M. Ward, and J. Nwokike. 2018. Expanding global access to essential medicines: Investment priorities for sustainably strengthening medical product regulatory systems. *Global Health* 14(1):102.

Ruger, J. P. 2007. Global health governance and the World Bank. *The Lancet* 370 (9597):1471–1474.

Teo, H. S. 2016. *Medicines regulatory systems and scope for regulatory harmonization in Southeast Asia.* Washington, DC: The World Bank Group.

UN (United Nations). 2018. *Countries urged to strengthen tax systems to promote inclusive economic growth.* New York: United Nations Department of Economic and Social Affairs. https://www.un.org/development/desa/en/news/financing/tax4dev.html (accessed July 30, 2019).

UNODC (United Nations Office on Drugs and Crime). n.d. *Model laws and treaties.* https://www.unodc.org/unodc/en/legal-tools/model-treaties-and-laws.html (accessed November 13, 2019).

Vapnek, J., and M. Spreij. 2005. *Perspectives and guidelines on food legislation, with a new model food law.* Rome, Italy: Development Law Service FAO Legal Office.

WBG (The World Bank Group). 2018a. Global indicators of regulatory governance full data 2018. Washington, DC: The World Bank Group.

WBG. 2018b. *Worldwide governance indicators.* https://info.worldbank.org/governance/wgi/#home (accessed July 26, 2019).

Whitmore Schanzenbach, D., R. Nunn, L. Bauer, and M. Mumford. 2016. *Where does all the money go: Shifts in household spending over the past 30 years.* Washington, DC: The Hamilton Project.

WHO (World Health Organization). 1999. *Marketing authorization of pharmaceutical products with special reference to multisource (generic) products: A manual for drug regulatory authorities.* http://apps.who.int/medicinedocs/en/d/Js2273e/12.html (accessed February 13, 2020).

WHO. 1999. *Annex 8: National drug regulatory legislation: Guiding principles for small drug regulatory authorities.* Geneva, Switzerland: WHO.

WHO. 2014. *Regulatory system strengthening for medical products.* http://apps.who.int/medicinedocs/documents/s21456en/s21456en.pdf (accessed April 29, 2019).

WHO. 2017. Food safety and nutrition food law guidelines. Brazzaville, Congo: WHO Regional Office for Africa. https://www.afro.who.int/publications/food-safety-and-nutrition-food-law-guidelines (accessed August 8, 2019).

WHO. 2018a. WHO Global Benchmarking Tool (GBT) for evaluation of national regulatory system of medical products. In *National Regulatory System (RS): Indicators and Fact Sheets.* Geneva, Switzerland: WHO. https://www.who.int/medicines/areas/regulation/01_GBT_RS_RevVI.pdf?ua=1 (accessed July 26, 2019).

WHO. 2018b. *WHO Global Benchmarking Tool (GBT) for evaluation of national regulatory system of medical products: Glossary and definitions revision VI version 1*. Geneva, Switzerland: WHO.

WHO EMRO (Eastern Mediterraean Regional Office). n.d. *Global health needs global health diplomacy*. http://www.emro.who.int/health-topics/health-diplomacy/about-health-diplomacy.html (accessed November 7, 2019).

World Bank. n.d.-a. *Global indicators of regulatory governance*. https://rulemaking.worldbank.org (accessed September 9, 2019).

World Bank. n.d.-b. *Transparency of rulemaking*. https://rulemaking.worldbank.org/en/data/comparedata/transparency (accessed September 9, 2019).

5

The Role of the Regulatory Agency

The two previous chapters in this report considered distal influences on the regulatory system: actions at the global level that can encourage product safety and how decisions made at higher levels of government can affect the ability of the regulatory agency to function. This chapter considers tasks that are, for the most part, within the control of decision makers at the regulatory agency. It also sets out some principles regulators can use to ensure their invariably limited resources are being deployed efficiently.

The strategies put forth in this chapter aim to increase the scientific credibility and efficiency of regulatory agencies. Risk is the best guiding principle to lead the agency to this goal. Chapter 2 described the continuous risk management cycle through which agencies are constantly identifying risks and ranking the risks of varying complexity and certainty (IOM and NRC, 2010a). This chapter discusses a range of risks facing regulatory agencies, especially in low- and middle-income countries, as well as strategies to mitigate these risks.

STRATEGIES FOR MANAGING RISK

A 2010 report from the Institute of Medicine and the National Research Council, *Enhancing Food Safety: The Role of the Food and Drug Administration*, set out the attributes of a risk-based food safety system (see Box 5-1), all of which are sufficiently general that they apply to medical products as well. Reliable data are part of such a system, as is the technical depth at the agency to make good use of data. Without reliable and accurate data, shared promptly and through secure means, no agency can

BOX 5-1
Attributes of a Risk-Based System

A risk-based system is proactive and based on a strategic management plan. Notwithstanding the need to respond to unforeseeable crises, risk activities should be planned in advance, an exercise that should include various stakeholders and be based on the knowledge gained from past experience with a vision of predicting food contamination problems. Managing a crisis in the short term and implementing a well-developed strategic plan for managing food safety in the long term are equally important; attention to unanticipated outbreaks should not detract from implementation of the strategic plan.

A risk-based system is data driven. Although expert opinion is a valuable asset when there are uncertainties or data must be interpreted, a risk-based system should be grounded in science. That is, the collection, analysis, and interpretation of quality data, as well as data management, are essential tasks for the implementation of a risk-based system.

A risk-based system is grounded in the principles of risk analysis. A risk-based system should be grounded in risk analysis, with risk assessment, risk communication, and risk management as the essential basis for establishing a sound public health protection capability. If implemented appropriately, the system ideally provides a transparent, data-driven means by which to determine the extent of public health protection achieved as a result of different risk management actions, and therefore it provides a decision-making tool. This concept has worldwide support and has been applied for several decades by regulatory and public health agencies.

A risk-based system employs analytical methods to rank risks based on public health impact. A risk-based system systematically ranks risks even if those risks differ in complexity and uncertainty. The development of analytical methods (models) that can assign numerical values to the various risks based on public health impact is the foundation of this activity.

A risk-based system employs analytical methods to prioritize the allocation of limited resources to manage risk most effectively. The evaluation of intervention strategies is an essential element of risk management. Risk managers must consider multiple characteristics or attributes of different risks and integrate these data for the purpose of prioritizing and making effective use of resources. In this manner, decisions are made by considering the food system as a whole, that is, with a systems-based approach. Important decision analysis tools that may be used in this process are feasibility, cost-effectiveness, and cost-benefit analyses. A major element of this activity is a clear statement of regulatory philosophy and the use of a road map showing how decisions will be made regarding the mix of private responsibility, government incentives, and government regulation that will be used to manage different risks.

A risk-based system considers other factors, such as consumer perception, cost, controllability, public acceptance, environmental effects, and market impacts, in decision making when appropriate. Risk mitigation strategies and public policy decision making are influenced by factors other than public health risk. These considerations should be formally communicated to stakeholders.

A risk-based system employs measures to evaluate the efficacy of the risk management program on a continuous basis. An essential step in a risk-based system is evaluation of the efficacy of the system itself with respect to public health and other factors selected by decision makers. Evaluation of programs, always a daunting process, requires the identification of indicators by which to link interventions to public health outcomes. To collect and integrate food safety data so that attribution models can be built is a critical first step in this process.

A risk-based system performs all of these functions in a systematic and transparent manner with the involvement of stakeholders. Risk managers should develop a process for implementing a two-way communication approach whereby stakeholders have an opportunity to engage in the risk-based decision-making process. This approach should include input and access to discussions regarding the basis for decision making, as well as information about the uncertainties and variability of the underlying data. Likewise, a risk-based approach requires disclosure of all sources of information, comprehensive analysis, and transparency regarding the considerations taken into account in the decision-making process. In addition, independent peer review is fundamental to all scientific undertakings and critical for risk-based, decision-making processes.

SOURCE: IOM and NRC, 2010b.

understand the risks facing it or even begin the iterative process of risk ranking and intervention.

At the same time, the committee recognizes that an over-emphasis on the ideal risk analysis can be a barrier to progress in low- and middle-income countries. In reality, decisions on how to reduce risks, even at the most advanced agencies, are made in the face of uncertainty. When time or resources are constraints, a narrative or qualitative risk analysis may be the best strategy (Paoli, 2010). While the inferences drawn from narrative or even semi-quantitative data are not as strong as probabilistic inferences, less quantitative assessments can be done faster and at lower cost (Paoli, 2010).

Therefore, risk-based approaches are appropriate in low- and middle-income countries' regulatory agencies, recognizing that the perfect need not be the enemy of the good. While acknowledging that the public sector is often limited in its data and capacity for analysis, regulators can still use a risk-based approach to understanding and making use of the information they have.

Furthermore, the risk-based framework, even when applied with imperfect data, draws attention to the relative vulnerabilities in a country's system (Babigumira et al., 2018). Understanding these weak spots is essential for the proportional allocation of resources that helps countries transition off donor funding (Babigumira et al., 2018).

Some evidence suggests that the risks facing a country will vary with economic development. For example, increasing income and urbanization bring about new risks as the distance between farm and table grows and diets become more diverse (Jaffee et al., 2019). Microbial contamination, for example, is more of a problem as people eat more animal-source foods requiring refrigeration; as people take more meals outside the home they are exposed to more and different food-handling risks (Jaffee et al., 2019). Different populations within a country can face different risks, especially in middle-income countries, which bear a dual burden of naturally occurring hazards, such as mycotoxins, and those associated with modernizing systems and increased processing, such as microbial and chemical contamination (Jaffee et al., 2019). In considering the medicines market, the relative openness of a country's borders can affect the risk of falsified or substandard medicines in its market (Babigumira et al., 2018).

Effective Use of Data

The effective use of data is a critical bottleneck to agencies' scientific rigor and risk-based decision making (IOM, 2012). Part of the challenge in collecting data is knowing how to monitor the market; not all product safety events are equally important to the regulatory agency. In considering how to collect data, it is important to identify risks that occur frequently enough to produce data; events where past risks are predictive of the future, making them useful for predictive modeling; and where a baseline may be established. Information about foodborne disease outbreaks, inspection reports, and records of previous regulatory action such as recalls would meet these criteria. There are also questions of access, if, for example, data will be entered manually or pulled from automated sources. An important first step to better information management is for the agency to take stock of the data produced in its routine monitoring programs and to assess its usefulness. Then, if necessary, the agency can consider various strategies to improve the data available. For example, 2018 guidance from the Promoting the Quality of Medicines program made the distinction between sporadic quality surveys of medicines in the market, and a predictable, strategic post-market surveillance system (Kaddu et al., 2018).

Epidemiological data are useful for regulatory agencies. They are a direct measure of public health consequences, and there are often at least nascent systems in place to collect it (WHO, 2017b). Expressing health outcomes in terms of quality or disability-adjusted life years allows for valid comparisons to other health programs (Babigumira et al., 2018). At the same time, links between epidemiological data and regulatory problems can be tenuous at best. Foodborne illness in particular is under-reported, even in places with sophisticated surveillance and reporting systems (Jaffee et al., 2019). In the case of poor quality medicines, the relationship between a death or illness and a contaminated product may be even more obscure as medicines are usually given to people who are already sick, clouding the relationship between cause and effect (IOM, 2013).

Over the last few years, the analysis of big data (the large amounts of data produced in digital interactions) has been promoted for its promise to improve health and livelihoods around the world (Bresnick, 2019; Raghupathi and Raghupathi, 2014; Serra, 2016). Big data, which includes information drawn from manufacturing, health services, business, and government agencies (to name a few), has particular promise for low- and middle-income countries, where even estimating the scope of food and medicine safety problems is a challenge (Serra, 2016; Wyber et al., 2015). Most vertical health programs collect considerable information from health workers (Wyber et al., 2015); manufacturing and government records are similarly rich in data.

The promise of technology to reduce the cost of aggregating and collecting data is especially valuable when resources are scarce. In a joint statement on food safety and trade, the Food and Agriculture Organization of the United Nations (FAO), the World Health Organization (WHO), and the World Trade Organization (WTO) praised the promise of big data to facilitate trade, improve traceability and safety, and allow the food system to respond to various threats (FAO et al., 2019). Savings on transaction costs add up, especially for perishable food. A 1 percent savings on transaction costs, when magnified over the supply chain, yields a benefit of $43 billion (FAO et al., 2019). But realizing these benefits requires cooperation within and among countries, as well as cooperation with the private sector and academia (FAO et al., 2019).

Data sharing is an intermediary on the way to realizing the potential of big data. Research on data sharing in low- and middle-income countries is promising; for the most part, scientists support data sharing to advance science and collaboration, as well as for networking and visibility (Bezuidenhout and Chakauya, 2018). This is consistent with the emerging global consensus in favor of data sharing, though this consensus has yet to translate into widespread practice (Bezuidenhout and Chakauya, 2018; Cheah, 2019; Waithira et al., 2019). In places where reliable electricity, connection speed, and processing power cannot be taken for granted, support for data sharing or big data can seem overly ambitious (Bezuidenhout and Chakauya, 2018). Because of problems with management and weak health systems (of which the regulatory system is just one part) the promise of modern data analytics has remained out of reach in low- and middle-income countries (Wyber et al., 2015). The irony of the problem remains: When food and drug safety problems are more common, the tools to understand them are more valuable, but scarce (Waithira et al., 2019). Despite growing support for data sharing, there are "few incentives and multiple barriers" to its implementation (Hajduk et al., 2019). The main obstacles to data sharing in low- and middle-income countries, especially for regulatory agencies, are not clear and may be a question for the proposed Centers of Excellence in Regulatory Science (Bezuidenhout and Chakauya, 2018). Research in the United States has found data governance to be the biggest barrier (Poole and Harpel, 2018). It is also possible that the mechanism for data sharing (e.g., the use of automated collection systems or secure online sharing) may be an important barrier in less developed countries. Box 5-2 describes a program that aims to remove such barriers for clinical trials researchers in sub-Saharan Africa.

The private sector is often reluctant to share data; they may fear that information in their internal reports introduce liability or damage their reputation (Narrod et al., 2019b). Concerns about the direct costs associated with data sharing are also common (Narrod et al., 2019a,b). Blinding or aggregating data, possibly with a university or other trusted third-party acting as intermediary, is one way around this barrier (Narrod et al., 2019a).

Another common barrier when sharing information with the private sector is a company policy at odds with that of the regulatory agency. For example, pharmaceutical companies often have their own teams investigate reports of falsified and substandard medicines (Access to Medicine Foundation, 2018). Companies are obliged to confirm cases and report them

BOX 5-2
The Knowledge Hub for Clinical Trial Data Sharing

The European and Developing Countries Clinical Trials Partnership is a source for guidance and training on how to manage data in a way that facilitates its sharing. Working with the Global Health Network, an online platform for researchers in global health, the partnership has created a repository that provides guidance on all aspects of working with and sharing health data. This repository, called a "knowledge hub," has resources such as a tool kit on data sharing, including an online tool to navigate various data repositories, and an overview of the steps in data sharing. The tool kit gives detailed examples of important documents, such as patient consent forms that allow for sharing research data. It also explains the different models for access to the data (open, controlled, or closed) and different strategies to organize and name files.

The courses, protocols, and guidelines available through the knowledge hub have been designed for clinical trials data but are widely applicable to other health data. The project is also new, and some aspects such as the data management resources were still in development when this report was published. Nevertheless, the concrete steps given can make the process of data sharing and the front-end management work that facilitates such sharing more manageable. As of 2018, 194 African research centers were participating in the European and Developing Countries Clinical Trials Partnership, with particular success in developing medicines, diagnostics, and other tools to fight infectious disease in sub-Saharan Africa. Facilitating data sharing among these researchers is an important step in support of a global public good.

SOURCES: EDCTP, n.d.; EDCTP Knowledge Hub, n.d.-a, n.d.-b; Hajduk et al., 2019; The Global Health Network, 2019.

to the local regulatory authority or to the WHO within 7 days (Access to Medicine Foundation, 2018). Nevertheless, a 2018 survey of 20 large firms found that only 35 percent followed these guidelines (Access to Medicine Foundation, 2018).

Regulatory agencies should give special attention to their data policies (Waithira et al., 2019). This includes the models they will use (options range from online open databases to managed access via application), their confidentiality restrictions, and processes for resolving disputes (Poole and Harpel, 2018; Waithira et al., 2019; Wyber et al., 2015). Clarity regarding the rules for data sharing can encourage more stakeholders to be comfortable with it, ultimately building relationships, especially with the industry stakeholders whose participation is vital (Poole and Harpel, 2018). At the same time, there are circumstances where industry representatives will object to information sharing because of confidentiality concerns. It is important to provide industry with both reasons for sharing and a motivation to do so (Narrod et al., 2019b). Regulators can prepare for a potential conflict by highlighting in the data-sharing policy their standards for public transparency, making clear that the health of the public takes precedence over any commercial interests.

Scarce resources are valuable, and data used to monitor food and medical product safety can be scarce, especially for regulatory agencies. Data sharing can help overcome this scarcity. The U.S. Office of Management and Budget's recent direction to heads of agencies and departments framed data sharing and management as stewardship of the taxpayers' money, encouraging them to harness existing information to answer policy questions (Vought, 2019). This first step in this process may be taking stock of which other agencies or private-sector organizations might already have the information they need, and if they are willing to share it. When food safety responsibilities are divided between the ministries of health and agriculture, as in the United States, a strategy for cooperation can help avoid redundant work and maximize the value of information. Businesses also collect valuable information from across their supply chains, information that would help regulators identify potential risks and areas to concentrate their resources (Harkins, 2016). As Malcolm Harkins explained in *Managing Risk and Information Security*, "Because threats spread so quickly and the threat landscape is so complex, it is hard for any single organization to gain a clear view of all potential vulnerabilities, threats, and attacks. External partnerships can help. They provide additional intelligence that we can use to improve our [security]" (Harkins, 2016).

But sharing sensitive information is difficult for all parties. Public–private partnerships can be effective means for data sharing (Narrod et al., 2019b). Novel information-sharing technologies, though not a substitute for building trust, also have potential to help overcome this problem (Knowledge@Wharton, 2018).

Distributed Ledger Technology

Distributed ledger technologies (of which blockchain is one type) are databases that are synchronized across different computers, with certain participants in the system having the authority to update the entire network (Pisa and McCurdy, 2019). Systems can be described as either permissioned or permission-less, depending on the authorization for updating them (Pisa and McCurdy, 2019). These databases hold more information, more securely than other data management systems (Verhoeven et al., 2018). And, because there is no central database or single person in charge of the system, the administrative costs of collecting and managing data are greatly reduced (Verhoeven et al., 2018).

Distributed ledgers have particular promise for managing complicated supply chains. Tracing ingredients through a supply chain could allow for quick pinpointing of where contamination occurs; it could be used to verify label claims, or to better understand patterns of supply and demand, helping procurement officers avoid shortages or waste (Pisa and McCurdy, 2019). But there are still questions as to what range of network sophistication lends itself to distributed ledgers (Knowledge@Wharton, 2018). Experts have cautioned against the overuse or novelty appeal of such technology, especially in low- and middle-income countries where the cost of distraction could be high (Knowledge@Wharton, 2018). At the same time, the IBM Food Trust is using blockchain technology to allow farmers, processors, or any food supplier to share data with their networks (IBM, 2019; Knowledge@Wharton, 2018). Through the use of an online app that feeds into a blockchain system, farmers can send information about their produce to buyers, reducing the time needed to trace a supply chain from about a week to seconds (Knowledge@Wharton, 2018).

The realities of modern manufacturing have made supply chain traceability a priority for regulatory agencies around the world, but traceability programs produce massive amounts of data that can be difficult to manage (Pisa and McCurdy, 2019). It is important to set the groundwork now to make use of those data. An investment in data and their management will pay off in better knowledge of vulnerabilities in the supply chain and information on waste, surplus, supply, and demand. (Box 5-3 describes how advanced data analytics helped the U.S. Department of Agriculture target its food inspections.) These are the same data that inform procurement and should therefore be especially high priority in the middle-income countries projected to graduate from multilateral procurement over the next 20 years (Pisa and McCurdy, 2019; Silverman, 2018).

Assessing Health and Economic Effects of Regulation

A strong regulatory system protects public health and also has positive spillovers for the economy. A poorly designed system obviously has disastrous implications for health; it can also lower growth, create market confusion, and reduce competition. Nevertheless, estimating these effects is challenging. There are many intermediaries between a good regulatory practice, say public consultation on rules, and gross domestic product growth (Parker and Kirkpatrick, 2012). Even measuring the health effects is not direct. Except in crises, when a product safety failure has caused obvious illness or worse, it is difficult to say what portion of health improvement or economic growth can be credibly attributed to the regulatory

BOX 5-3
Risk-Based Inspections

The U.S. Department of Agriculture's Food Safety and Inspection Service implemented a sampling plan in 2007 that produced more informative data and allowed the agency to better target its resources. The agency's new plan was a risk-based algorithm that categorized the risk of different types of facilities, making the type of inspection required a function of that risk. It also gave more attention to higher risk animal-source foods, such as meat, poultry, and eggs.

To determine which establishments pose the greatest risk, the agency built the Public Health Information System to collect, consolidate, and analyze data from inspections and food safety assessments. Having high-quality data led to the development of new policies, sampling and inspection procedures, and enhanced performance measurement. To ensure the consistency and quality of data, the agency formed the Data Analysis and Integration Group and the Data Coordination Committee to oversee the processes. They are responsible for ensuring consistency and coordinating all data collection and analysis.

The agency will also use the data to modernize inspection procedures. For example, to improve analysis capabilities during inspections, early warning alerts are set up and data regarding food safety concerns are delivered to inspectors in real-time. Providing high-quality data at the first sign of non-compliance can encourage prompt corrective action and reduce non-compliance.

SOURCES: USDA, 2010a,b, 2016; USDA and Office of Inspector General, 2007.

system. This presents a dilemma for regulators, because that is precisely the analysis that would be most compelling to their ministers.

There is a time lag between a regulatory policy going into effect and measurable changes taking place (Narrod et al., 2019b). Analysis of the casual chain between a policy and its health or other effects is one tool to overcome this gap (Parker and Kirkpatrick, 2012). Cost-benefit analysis—the estimating of direct and indirect costs and benefits associated with regulatory policies—can be helpful (Parker and Kirkpatrick, 2012). The problem remains, however, that the technical skill to perform such economic evaluations will not always be available in-house at a regulatory agency. The proposed Centers of Excellence in Regulatory Science could take on these analyses when necessary. The regulatory agency can also facilitate good analysis by clearly stating in the goal of regulatory policy the evidence that will be evaluated and sources of this evidence, as well as indicating how the effects of a policy might influence various subpopulations (Jessup, 2013). Organisation for Economic Co-operation and

Development (OECD) guidance on Regulatory Impact Analysis will be a valuable resource in setting up such assessment, as is the U.S. government primer on the topic (OECD, n.d.-b; Office of Information and Regulatory Affairs, 2011). Useful examples of such analyses can also be found on the U.S. Food and Drug Administration (FDA) website (FDA, 2019).

Public–private partnerships are another important means to build capacity for food and medicine safety; such partnerships have potential to ease data sharing and build trust among various partners. The Asia-Pacific Economic Cooperation's Partnership Training Institute Network involves regulators and private sector participants in trainings to advance a shared goal of improving food safety (APEC, 2018). The World Bank's Global Food Safety Partnership (GFSP) also brings together government, industry, and academic experts to build capacity for food safety (GFSP, n.d.). GFSP and the United Nations Industrial Development Organization recently began an extensive capacity building program for managing downstream food suppliers in Asia, Africa, and the Middle East (UNIDO, 2016). Research pharmaceutical companies are also increasingly involved in capacity building and in partnerships for research in low- and middle-income countries, with the goal of increasing access to medicines (Hogerzeil et al., 2014; Stevens et al., 2017).

Communication

A unique challenge facing regulatory agencies is that their job, when done well, is invisible. Effective medicines are not praised in stemming an outbreak any more than a restaurant critic would laud food for being uncontaminated. In the inevitable balancing against other flashier pieces of the health system, the regulatory agency stands to lose. For this reason, regulators need to advocate the importance of their work—to their ministers, to industry, and to the public. It is difficult during quiet times to explain to these audiences why support for regulatory agencies is so important. Therefore, crises present an important opportunity for education and advocacy.

Classically characterized by "a threat, a short decision time, and surprise," more modern definitions of crisis emphasize a threat "to the basic structures or fundamental values of a system" (Boin et al., 2005; Hermann, 1969). By either definition, crises affecting food and medical products have hit all countries in the last decade, raising fundamental questions about the adequacy of government regulatory efforts. Contaminated spinach, toothpaste, blood thinners, infant formula, peanut products, and compounded medicines have raised alarm in the United States and abroad (Andrews, 2012; Bloomberg News, 2019; Browne, 2018; Greenemeier, 2008; Harris, 2006; Reuters, 2007). Other crises are based more on fear than actual evidence of harm, as when the FDA had to address the safety of apple juice after low, naturally occurring levels of arsenic were identified (Anderson, 2011).

There are serious economic consequences to product safety crises that reach the level of a recall. Grocery Manufacturers Association estimates put the direct cost of a food recall around $10 million to the company alone (Ostroff, 2018). Estimates of the cost of medical product recalls are harder to come by, but a recent study by McKinsey & Company found that medical device recalls could cost a company between $250 and $600 million (Fuhr et al., 2013). Such estimates do not even begin to account for the cost to a company's reputation or to the damage to markets wrought by loss of confidence in public institutions.

Product safety crises offer a chance to strengthen regulatory infrastructure. The distinction between the sort of crisis that undermines the agency and that which causes people to rally behind it are not always clear, but it seems that strong, effective public communication can make the difference between an embarrassing debacle and grateful support for the agency. For example, when an antimicrobial agent called the Elixir Sulfanilamide was found to be contaminated in 1937, the FDA sent inspectors across the country to track down and dispose of the dangerous product. Instead of blaming the FDA for letting the crisis happen in the first place, the public cheered the agency's dogged pursuit of risky medication. Momentum from the agency's success led to the passage of the Food, Drug, and Cosmetic Act the next year (Sharfstein, 2018).

Effective communication during a crisis requires preparation. The U.S. Centers for Disease Control and Prevention's Crisis and Emergency Risk Communications manual sets out a series of capabilities needed for accomplishing these goals effectively (CDC, 2014). The FAO has a similar handbook for communicating food risks (FAO and WHO, 2016). Key principles include understanding the audience and the stress the crisis situation has wrought as well as simple, honest messages, including a frank assessment of any uncertainty (CDC, 2014; FAO and WHO, 2016). It is important that crisis communication start as soon as the problem becomes evident, with trained staff clearly and publicly explaining what is known and unknown about the situation, ideally including concrete recommendations as to how people can protect themselves.

Social media are an important route for these communications. Agencies can participate in popular social networks, such as Twitter, with accounts designed for information about recalls and other emergencies. The FDA Twitter account @FDArecalls is an example of such an account (FDA, 2008). Agencies should also respond to misinformation on social media within the same channel, so that someone who sees misleading information on Facebook, for example, can access the correct information from the agency on the same site.

Crises present a unique opportunity because they bring a spotlight onto the regulatory agency. The tragedy of the product safety failure is only compounded if the agency fails to use that spotlight as impetus for change. For example, in 2010 there was a *salmonella* outbreak from contaminated eggs in the United States (CDC, 2010). FDA leaders, by virtue of careful preparation and knowledge of their risks, were able to segue the attention from the outbreak into support for the Food Safety Modernization Act (Sharfstein, 2018). Internal preparation, and continued, ongoing communication regarding the risks facing the agency can help an agency's leaders prepare for such a situation.

An agency's crisis communication plan is, in many ways, an outgrowth of its routine communication. An outreach strategy during an outbreak must start from a routine communication strategy, drawing on existing relationships. Routine communication on the agency's work, through public consultations, for example, encourages connection with industry and with private citizens (OECD, 2016, n.d.-a; WBG, 2010). Regulators need to recognize the value of public consultations by responding to comments received and explaining the rationale for accepting or rejecting them (OECD, 2016). Such ordinary communication creates a culture of openness that is even more important given the challenges of misleading information circulating via the Internet and social media.

The Internet and social media are invaluable for outreach and education, both critical responsibilities of the regulatory agency. Agencies now have access to a wide range of tools to inform the public about everything from how to cook a chicken safely to where to file an adverse event report. These different platforms are important to integrated health promotion strategies, as is coordination with other public health agencies. Agencies can also choose to receive information from the public through text messages, Twitter, and other platforms. Such communication has a democratizing effect on both knowledge and engagement.

At the same time, social media can be a vehicle for misinformation (Meserole, 2018). Agencies are increasingly called upon to combat such misinformation and may need to work through the same networks spreading the falsehoods (Jaffee et al., 2019; Larson, 2018; Lau et al., 2012).

Furthermore, a great deal of regulatory work is highly technical and complicated, itself a barrier to public appreciation for it. Good manufacturing practices, critical control points, and quality specifications are not usually defined in ways that are easy to understand. As a result, the media, legislators, and the public may not appreciate the need for greater investment in the regulatory agency as a way to protect and promote health.

Given the challenges currently affecting regulatory agencies, it is necessary to re-evaluate the risks facing them. When regulators do this, they should give particular attention to the data systems that help them manage risks, the work they share with international partners, building internal capacity, and communication.

Recommendation 5-1: National regulatory authorities should take a risk-based approach to the regulation of food and medicines. This includes:

- **a. Developing effective data systems to systematically identify areas of greatest risk;**
- **b. Participating in research, data-sharing, technology adoption, and training activities with international partners;**
- **c. Growing capacity to assess the health and economic impacts of regulation, and using this information to inform actions to protect public health;**
- **d. Communicating about risks, including the uncertainty around them, especially during a crisis; and**
- **e. Communicating the ways regulation improves quality, safety, and access, using different strategies to convey this information to government leaders, regulated industry, and the public.**

Every agency has to make different determinations about the risks confronting it; those determinations are based both on data and on an understanding of the will of society. To this end, every agency needs access to information and a strategy to communicate with government leaders, the public, and regulated industry, both to solicit their input and to convey the risks facing the agency.

Identifying and ranking risks depend on data and analytic skills. For this reason, the WHO Global Benchmarking Tool is designed with subindicators in each of the nine key functions relating to risk management. Analysis of these indictors can give some insight into an agency's ability to identify and rank the risks facing it (WHO, n.d.). The WHO and the FAO Food Control System Assessment Tool also emphasizes "capacity to collect and analyze data for risk analysis" (Caipo, 2019). As more countries undergo these assessments, it may be possible to say with more precision how many regulatory agencies can properly use risk to inform decision making.

Furthermore, neither frank communication with the public nor crisis management is easy in places where there is not a certain level of media openness or diversity of sources (OECD, 2016). Nonetheless, effective communication is essential to garnering the support necessary for the regulatory mission. Most regulatory agencies can use cases where serious harm has been averted to their advantage. One famous instance of harm averted is the FDA's denial of market authorization to thalidomide in the 1960s (FDA, 2018b). There are many examples from low- and middle-income countries as well. For example, in 2017, the Tanzania Food and Drug Authority began a program of soliciting reports of suspicious products from doctors, pharmacists, and other health workers using smartphones. The successful implementation of this program led to the recall of substandard malaria diagnostic kits (WHO, 2017a).

More mundane regulatory work is also an opportunity for communication. The Food Safety and Standards Authority of India's webpage Success Stories, for example, advertises the agency's work, including programs to improve the safety of street food (FSSAI, n.d.). Press releases, website announcements, blogs, and smartphone apps are all channels the agency can use to reach the public with messages about the value of newly approved medicines or seasonal food safety warnings. There is also value to publicizing more controversial actions the agency takes to protect public health, such as revocations of licenses or sanctions, before the aggrieved manufacturer does. Using a diversity of tools ensures a wider reach; it also helps the agency stay in control of competing narratives concerning regulatory action.

A good communication strategy considers the type of audience targeted, the tools used to reach them, and clarity of presentation. (Materials intended for health professionals, for example, are written at a different level than those meant for all parents of young children.) A plan to evaluate the effectiveness of the communication materials and areas for improvement should also be articulated early (FDA, n.d.). Such evaluations can measure how aware consumers are of the agency's work and how far its communications tools reach, especially considering reach in vulnerable communities. These evaluations can guide periodic reshaping of the communication strategy. For example, an evaluation of the FDA's system for reporting possible adverse events associated with prescription medicines found that posting on early signals may have increased alarm unnecessarily (Chakraborty and Lofstedt, 2012). Regulators may also need to assess this type of sentiment and reshape their strategies in response.

Information on the effects of regulatory action can be especially valuable. Box 5-4 describes how regulatory action can influence diet, for example. If developments at the regulatory agency stand to grow the economy, this too should be publicized. While acknowledging that the price of medicines is influenced by many factors, the agency should be willing to comment on its contribution to economic gains. In El Salvador, for example, revisions to the national medicines law made it easier for quality-approved generics to enter the market, contributing to a 20 to 25 percent reduction in the price of medicines (Yamagiwa, 2015). In Mexico, concerted attention to eliminating the application backlog greatly increased the number of registered generics between 2011 and 2016 and brought down the cost of medicines by about 50 percent on average (Arriola Penalosa et al., 2017).

BOX 5-4
Food Labeling and Child Obesity

Among those authorities traditionally granted to regulatory agencies is the authority to require businesses to label products, in a manner that is truthful and not misleading, as to contents, potential adverse effects, and hazards (e.g., alcoholic beverages, cigarettes). Advertising claims can be considered an extension of the label claims and therefore subject to regulation.

Obesity is a risk factor for chronic disease and is a good case study of how regulatory agencies can be part of broad public health campaigns in low- and middle-income countries. The global obesity epidemic affects the same countries dealing with infectious diseases and undernutrition, with undernutrition and obesity often co-existing in the same household. The World Health Organization's response to this problem has included a Global Strategy on Diet, Physical Activity and Health and subsequently a Global Action Plan for the Prevention and Control of Noncommunicable Diseases 2013–2020.

Food policy interventions to prevent childhood obesity have been adopted in at least 22 countries or regions and include national nutrition education efforts (i.e., dietary guidelines), school food policy, food and menu labeling, food marketing (i.e., advertising restrictions), and food pricing (i.e., taxing unhealthy food and/or subsidizing healthy food). Taken together, this set of policies aims to change consumer behavior and reinforce healthy eating. Several countries in Latin America have adopted policies to prevent obesity in children. For example, Mexico has placed excise taxes on sugar-sweetened beverages and energy-dense foods aimed to decrease consumption. Chile, similarly, has imposed requirements for front-of-package labels with easy to understand messages about sugar, saturated fat, sodium, and calorie counts. Research indicates that these labels influence parents in their purchase of food for children.

SOURCES: Gostin, 2018; Instituto Nacional de Salud Pública de México, 2016; Perez-Escamilla et al., 2017; WHO, 2014; Zhang et al., 2014.

Finally, in considering the risks facing the regulatory agency, decision makers would do well to remember the importance of organizational culture. A major risk to many agencies is the inability to retain technical staff (IOM, 2012; OECD, 2016). Incentives such as good work–life balance and a career ladder with advancement opportunities can go far to correct this problem, even if government salaries cannot compete with those of the private sector (OECD, 2016).

THE RISKS OF INFORMAL MARKETS[1]

Data sharing, capacity building, and regulatory cooperation programs all have promise to make regulators work more efficiently, but these tools are all most effective in dealing with the formal, orderly operations of known producers and distributors. In low- and middle-income countries, considerable sale of food and medical products happens outside such channels. These informal markets are often a risk to public health, but steps to mitigating such risk are challenging; regulatory sanctions are, almost by definition, not an effective deterrent to producers who operate outside of the formal market (Jaffee et al., 2019). In such cases, regulators may need to give more attention to strategies to drive consumer preference to the best feasible option and to increase the reach of safe, good-quality options in the market.

Informal Markets for Food

Informal food markets are important in low- and middle-income countries, accounting for about 80 percent of food sold, possibly more in sub-Saharan Africa (Jaffee et al., 2019; Roesel and Grace, 2014). Urbanization contributes to the importance of informal markets, as city dwellers cannot produce their own food. Poor consumers in cities are not likely to have refrigeration, making daily food shopping necessary (Resnick, 2017). The International Livestock Research Institute estimates that poor and middle-class consumers buy almost all their nutritionally dense, animal-source foods in informal markets (Grace, 2015a; ILRI, 2010b). Animal-source foods are important for health; they are also high risk for microbial contamination. Market conditions in informal retail and wholesale are often lacking in refrigeration; safe storage and handling are never assured (Grace, 2015a; Grace et al., 2014; Jaffee et al., 2019; WHO, 2006).

It is often difficult for governments to know how to handle informal food markets. Attempts to arrest and fine informal sellers, destroy their marketplaces, or confiscate their wares are not uncommon, especially in Africa (Resnick, 2017). Such measures can have disastrous consequences for food security and livelihoods; it is not clear that they improve the underlying food safety problems either (Resnick, 2017). Enforcement alone is not likely to have any effect on the underlying market demand for the products informal sellers supply. Softer regulatory tools, such as consumer education, can help nudge consumer preference toward a safer alternative (Baldwin, 2014). Steps to professionalize the management of informal

[1] In this discussion, informal markets refers to "markets which escape effective health and safety regulation" (ILRI, n.d.).

markets can be helpful. For example, informal food markets in Zambia are managed by boards composed of consumers, vendors, and local authorities (Abrahams, 2009; Resnick, 2017). Involving vendors in the management of the markets made them more amenable to paying market fees to improve market sanitation (Abrahams, 2009; Resnick, 2017).

Research across a range of low- and middle-income countries has found consumers to be aware of the risks of microbial contamination in animal-source foods and produce (Alcorn and Ouyang, 2012; Grace, 2015a; ILRI, 2010b; Lapar and Toan, 2010). As a result, the demand for safer foods in domestic markets is predicted to grow over the next 20 years, as the middle class expands and education levels rise (Ortega and Tschirley, 2017). It is not clear what actions would increase consumer demand in such markets, however, or how consumer preferences affect producers (Ortega and Tschirley, 2017). One role for food regulators is to encourage demand for safety and to inform consumers about steps they can take to minimize the risks facing them.

On average, consumers in low- and middle-income countries are willing to pay a modest premium (by some estimates about 5 to 15 percent more) for safe foods (Roesel and Grace, 2014). Education and experience may influence willingness to pay. Research in rural Kenya found that shoppers who understood the danger of aflatoxins were willing to pay a higher premium for maize labeled "clean [of aflatoxin] and tested" (De Groote et al., 2016). This is consistent with research indicating the willingness to pay comes mostly from cities and wealthier shoppers; it increases with rising income, education, and exposure to media (Grace, 2015b; ILRI, 2010a,c; Ortega and Tschirley, 2017). It stands to reason that consumer education mass media are a necessary part of any food safety strategy (Morse et al., 2018). *The Safe Food Imperative* emphasized the role for consumer engagement, including education toward understanding various food quality indicators (Jaffee et al., 2019).

Evidence on the effectiveness of education to improve safe food practices at the level of farmers and food handlers is less clear (Grace et al., 2019; Jaffee et al., 2019). Although training can improve food safety in the short term, the benefits are not sustainable without continued institutional support (Grace et al., 2019). Since education alone does not necessarily transfer into safer food handling, strategies at the handling and processing levels can include certification or other measures to professionalize food handlers (Jaffee et al., 2019). There is also a role for research to identify methods that are effective for a given country's markets, bring them to scale, and adapt them to similar contexts. This is an area where the proposed Centers of Excellence in Regulatory Science could make useful contributions.

In most low- and middle-income countries, agriculture and food production are characterized by a great many small producers and large, informal markets complemented by a few very large firms; the structure of the market described sometimes as "elephants and mice" (Grace, 2015a). Given the logistical challenges of reaching all the players in informal food markets, it can be most efficient to introduce controls at aggregating points on the supply chain; the slaughterhouse, the dairy plant, and the wholesale market, for example (Grace et al., 2019). Other risks, such as chemical contamination from pesticides, are better managed at the farm (Jaffee et al., 2019). Working with small farmers on problems such as manure management and safe pesticide use are steps with health and environmental benefits even beyond food safety (Jaffee et al., 2019).

Informal Markets for Medicines

The informal medicines market is also a feature of medicine production and distribution in low- and middle-income countries, though less is known about its size or reach. Research from sub-Saharan Africa suggests that while pharmacies have good reach in cities, they are scarce in rural areas (Wafula et al., 2012). The vendors who operate in their stead are often not qualified for dispensing medicines, and the quality of the stock is uncertain (Wafula et al., 2012). Although the pharmacies in affluent, urban areas stock effective products, they charge accordingly, pricing out poor patients (Wafula et al., 2012). As with the informal food market, informal drug sellers meet a market demand for convenient and accessible sales at a low price (Goodman et al., 2007). And, as with foods, the poorest consumers are the ones most likely to use informal sellers (Bloom et al., 2014).

Regulatory agencies may be more likely to consider aggressive enforcement as a tool to shut down informal vendors in the medicines than food market, as there are not the same concerns about disrupting livelihoods. Closing illegal pharmacies and tightening control over the supply chain have been effective at reducing trade in falsified medicines in Rwanda and Cambodia (El-Jardali et al., 2015; Hamilton et al., 2016). It is not clear that this strategy is as effective in larger countries, however. After a series of raids on informal markets, warehouses, and shipments in the early 2000s, the Nigerian authorities concluded that the regulatory agency alone would not be able to put the informal sellers out of business (Chinwendu, 2008). More recent efforts to promote good distribution practices have promise to reduce the infiltration of falsified products into the supply chain; they also protect against accidental damage to good-quality products through inappropriate storage or handling (Fatokun, 2016; NAFDAC, 2016). Nevertheless, in Nigeria, as in many low- and middle-income countries, the large informal medicines market is a response to a demand for medicines that exceeds supply (NASEM, 2018). It is therefore necessary to increase the supply of affordable, good-quality alternatives.

The demand for medicines is predicted to grow, especially as countries move toward universal coverage (Pisani, 2019). By 2011 estimates, medicines accounted for two-thirds of government spending on health in some countries, a share that is only predicted to increase as the burden of paying for medicines slowly shifts from patients to governments (Lu et al., 2011; Pisani, 2019; Wagner et al., 2014). In the meantime, patients in much of the world will have to make purchasing decisions about medicines in a confusing market where the distinctions between good and bad quality are not clear.

Mobile technology used at the point of purchase can help motivated consumers verify the authenticity of products, usually by checking information on the package or by comparing a mobile photograph to an authentic image (Mackey and Nayyar, 2017). Such technology can be empowering to patients; it can also help engage the public in identifying breaches in the medicines supply chain (Mackey and Nayyar, 2017). For these reasons, the Nigerian regulatory authority is requiring mobile authentication on medicines packaging (PharmaSecure, n.d.); similar measures have been proposed in India (Sinha, 2011). Since the majority of adults in low- and middle-income countries have a mobile phone, these tools could be powerful (Dulli, 2019; Silver et al., 2019).

As in informal food markets, regulators have to use the tools available to them to direct consumers to the good-quality products and to educate society on the risks of shopping outside of regulated channels. Accreditation programs, as described in Box 5-5, hold particular promise for improving the reach of good-quality medical products.

Recommendation 5-2: National regulatory agencies should use evidence to guide strategies to reduce the risk posed by informal markets. Strategies to consider include accreditation or licensing to formalize sellers, consumer education, and increasing competition from regulated products.

In considering regulatory tools to combat informal markets, it is important to note what tools for change are realistically available to the regulatory agency. For instance, national price controls are not within the purview of the regulator, nor is the scope of the national medicines benefit package. A shortage of pharmacists might be remedied by task shifting, the process of delegating some to work to less trained staff, as described in Box 5-5. If professional practice laws disallow such shifts, however, the regulatory agency alone cannot change this. The role of the regulator is to improve access to safe, quality-assured products, but not to formalize the economy. Therefore, this recommendation is mainly concerned with ways

BOX 5-5
The Accredited Drug Dispensing Outlets in Tanzania

Informal medicines sellers are often popular in rural areas and other places pharmacies do not reach. Patients may value the convenience of the informal sellers, who are often an important source of health advice for communities. Recognizing the need these sellers meet, especially in underserved areas, the Tanzania Food and Drug Authority began an accreditation program in 2003. Over 9,000 drug stores have since been accredited, making the Accredited Drug Dispensing Outlets (ADDOs) the main medicines chain in Tanzania; 95 percent of Tanzanians live within 5 kilometers of an ADDO. The program has improved the quality and access to medicines, as well as rational use, including a particularly sharp improvement in observation of malaria treatment guidelines.

To gain accreditation, store owners and dispensing staff have to complete training in health, communication, and patient counseling, as well as local pharmacy laws, good dispensing practices, and rational use of medicines. The accreditation process also emphasizes business management skills, including record keeping. Review of ADDO records is, in turn, a window into dispensing practices and possible outbreaks for the health authorities. As an incentive to participate, shop owners are authorized to sell a limited list of restricted medicines, and the government promotes the stores through radio, flyers, and other mass media communication. Shop owners are also eligible for business improvement loans, allowing them to improve security or temperature control, for example. The program is also responsible for social benefits beyond those to health; as of 2013, about 90 percent of ADDO dispensing staff and 40 percent of owners are women.

One of the biggest advantages of the accreditation process is consolidated procurement. Pooled procurement means the store owners pay less for wholesale inventory; it also puts one qualified district-level officer in charge of wholesale purchases, a notoriously weak link in the drug supply chain. Improved procurement is reflected in the quality of the stock; over 90 percent of samples collected from ADDOs by secret shoppers passed quality testing. A different secret shopper study found that 90 percent of child pneumonia cases presented to ADDO staff were appropriately referred.

The ADDO model has been duplicated in Liberia and Uganda. Wider implementation is complicated, because the program can be in conflict with professional practice laws in some countries.

SOURCES: Chalker et al., 2015; Embrey et al., 2016; Kaale et al., 2016; Liana, 2014; MSH, 2013; Rutta, 2014.

to work with other actors in a decentralized system to encourage consumer behaviors that benefit health and stimulate a competitive market.

There is promise for market mechanisms to improve product safety in the food market, but the process will be slow (Jaffee et al., 2019). In the meantime, regulators have to choose their strategies to improve food safety in a way that promotes food security and rural livelihoods. Success depends a great deal on local context, making it difficult to identify transferable strategies (Grace, 2015a; Jaffee et al., 2019). The recent World Bank publication *The Safe Food Imperative* emphasized better engagement of consumers, tools to help consumers become "partners in food safety," and educational materials including education on understanding the various signals of quality in the markets, such as certification programs (Jaffee et al., 2019). Strategies that improve food safety should be inclusive to small farmers, many of whom are women who stand to lose in a rapid modernization of food systems (Grace, 2015a).

Translating food safety knowledge into behavior is often difficult (Zanin et al., 2017). Checklists can be a powerful tool for behavior change; sharing inspection checklists with food vendors, perhaps in simplified form, is one strategy to improve their observance of code (Jaffee et al., 2019). As with the informal medicines market, training and certification of vendors can help (FAO, 2016). Research in Kenya, India, and South Africa has shown that efforts to professionalize street vendors through a combination of training and incentives to be successful in improving food hygiene (FAO, 2016).

Consumer education is another invaluable tool for controlling risks of informal markets. The WHO's *Five Keys to Safer Foods* tool has been useful in reaching audiences from food vendors to home cooks and schoolchildren; it is available in 87 languages and has been used in 146 countries (Fontannaz-Aujoulat et al., 2019). Research in Cambodia, Ghana, and Vietnam has found the tool helpful in changing household and vendor behavior, Its success is often attributed to simple, clear messages, and explanations of the reasoning behind the behaviors promoted (Fontannaz-Aujoulat et al., 2019).

Education is a similarly important starting point for controlling informal medicines markets, described in a recent WHO report as, "the first step in preventing the use of substandard and falsified medicines" (WHO, 2017a). Anti-fraud packaging and point of use verification can help identify unsafe products at the point of purchase (Aminu et al., 2017; Hamilton et al., 2016), though these strategies may be most effective among fairly sophisticated consumers. Regulators may use media to direct business away from unlicensed vendors to safer ones, such as the accredited outlets described in Box 5-5. In choosing what strategies to promote, however, it is important to consider the agency's ability to follow through. Licensing vendors, for example, is not effective unless supported by inspection and enforcement tools (El-Jardali et al., 2015).

COOPERATION AT VARIOUS LEVELS

Steps taken to mitigate the risks of informal markets can be expected to have a disproportionate return to regulators in low- and middle-income countries because they depend on knowledge of local markets and local risks. Consumer education on safe food storage, for example, will be a successful strategy only if the messages are tailored to local problems and presented in a format accessible and salient to the intended audience. Activities where attention from the regulatory agency improves the safety of products on the market beyond the baseline comparison point should be priorities for regulatory agencies in low- and middle-income countries (Ahonkhai et al., 2016; Roth et al., 2018). The question that remains is how to manage the workload to enable regulators to devote more attention to the so-called value added activities.

Regulatory Reliance

The use of limited resources to add value requires prioritizing those tasks that elucidate risks, tasks such as market surveillance, inspecting distributors, and routine quality testing (Roth et al., 2018). There are also a great many regulatory responsibilities that do not pay off in terms of better understanding of local risks. These jobs are best approached with an eye toward maximizing efficiency and making use of the work of other, trusted organizations (OECD, 2018; Roth et al., 2018). For example, it is often prohibitively expensive to train staff to review new molecules in low- or middle-income countries, or even in many high-income ones. Since FDA or EMA approval is a global signal on the safety and efficacy of a new drug, it may be wise to defer these assessments (Moon et al., 2017). Staff time and funding can then be redirected to market surveillance (sometimes called "phase 4 studies") that clarify the risks of a drug in the population, adverse reactions, and interactions with other exposures (Cancer Research UK, 2019; HHS, n.d.).

Unilateral acceptance of the FDA or the EMA decisions is an example of regulatory reliance, the process by which an agency "take[s] into account or give[s] significant weight to work performed by another regulator or other trusted institution in reaching its own decision" (WHO, 2018). Reliance agreements allow authorities to make use of shared information, but retain the authority for regulatory decisions (Luigetti et al., 2016). Such reliance, especially in areas where a small agency's work adds little to no value, should be sought. Reliance agreements can be a boon to any agency looking to make more efficient use of available resources (Roth et al., 2018). Other benefits include improved scientific rigor, as decisions pull from more expertise and evidence; more opportunities for training and exchange; better clarity to regulated industry, which can encourage a more innovative private sector and a more predictable business environment; and increased networking with other regulatory experts.

Regulatory cooperation programs often draw on existing economic or political blocs, as in the East African Community and Association of Southeast Asian Nations examples mentioned in the previous chapter. Similarities in language or culture and existing trade relationships make these regional groupings obvious starting points for cooperation, but they need not be the only venue regulators pursue. As Figure 5-1 shows, there are a range of tools available for regulatory cooperation, some of which can be co-opted unilaterally (OECD, 2018; WHO, 2018). Unilateral reliance for some tasks can be a useful strategy while working on the longer-term goal of regional convergence (Roth et al., 2018).

Other Tools for Improving Efficiency

For most agencies, making good use of various tools for regulatory cooperation should be a priority. For some, this means taking advantage of

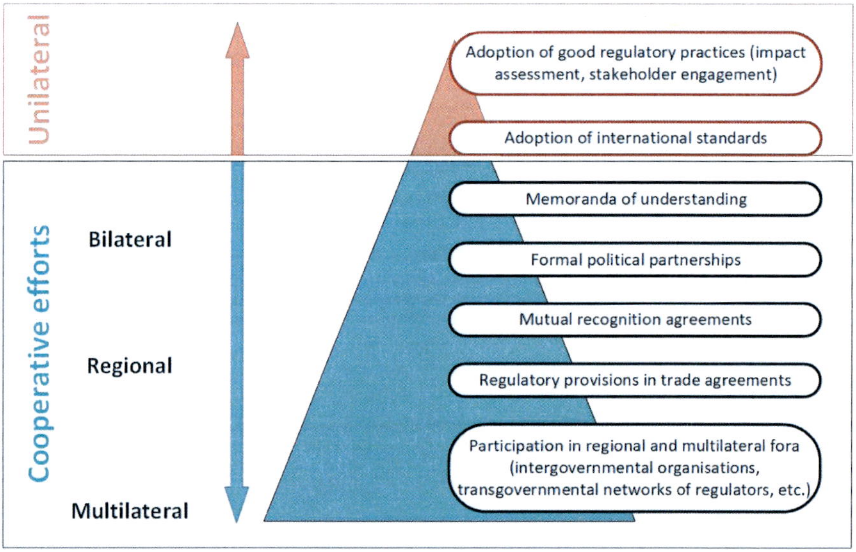

FIGURE 5-1 A continuum of tools for international regulatory cooperation.
SOURCES: OECD, 2018, based on OECD, 2013.

the work United Nations (UN) agencies do. The suggested expansion to the WHO prequalification program, recommended in Chapter 3, for example, is only meaningful if procurement agencies make use of the program. Reliance on prequalification saves national authorities time and money on dossier reviews, inspections, and other vetting of suppliers. Nonetheless, prequalified products still must be approved for use by each national regulatory authority, ensuring that registration being sought is for the identical product, dosage form, company, and manufacturer as the one listed with the WHO. The Collaborative Registration Procedure can ease the process of local registration for prequalified products and for products approved by advanced regulatory agencies[2] (WHO, 2016a,b). Since its launch in 2013, collaborative registration has expanded to over 30 countries (WHO, 2019). The program is also credited with significantly improving the registration process in participating countries; about half of collaborative registrations take 90 days or less (WHO, 2019).

Such cooperation with the WHO has tangible benefits to public health. When the WHO prequalified a meningococcal conjugate vaccine from Serum Institute of India, for example, it worked with regulatory authorities in Chad, Ethiopia, Ghana, Mali, Niger, Nigeria, and Senegal to introduce the vaccine, resulting in a roughly 90 percent reduction in risk of meningitis (Ahonkhai et al., 2016; Cooper et al., 2019; Daugla et al., 2014). The FAO and the WHO Codex Alimentarius Commission produces tools for food safety: Codex guidelines and standards are a good starting point for regulators looking to harmonize their national food laws (Halabi and Lin, 2017).

There are also a great many private organizations whose work can ease the task of regulatory cooperation. The International Council for Harmonisation of Technical Requirements for Pharmaceuticals for Human Use (ICH) produces technical guidelines to facilitate medicines registration, including a common format for regulatory review (ICH, n.d.). This format is now widely used, even in countries that are not ICH members, reducing unnecessary work for both government and industry (Garg et al., 2017).

Food regulation is arguably even more of a public–private operation, with certification now embedded into food laws in the United States, Europe, and parts of Asia (Halabi and Lin, 2017). The Euro-Retailer Produce Working Group protocol on good agricultural practices and the Global Food Safety Initiative standards discussed in Chapter 2 are other prominent examples of the so-called co-regulation of food safety, meaning a hybrid regulatory model with shared government and private sector responsibilities (Garcia Martinez et al., 2007). Table 5-1 shows how different types of food standards can be used by government or private-sector stakeholders.

[2] Meaning agencies benchmarked at level four, formerly described as "stringent regulatory agencies."

TABLE 5-1
Different Types of Public and Private Standards

Type of Standard	Source of Standard	Authority for Adoption	Implementation	Conformity Assessment	Enforcement	Examples
Regulations—Public, mandatory standards	Government	Legislation or regulatory agency	Private firms	Government inspector	Criminal or administrative courts	The regulatory authority's published rules
Public voluntary standards—Standards created by public bodies but whose adoption is voluntary	Government	Legislation or regulatory agency Private firms or organizations	Private firms	Auditor, can be government or private	Certification body; can be government or private	The French Ministry of Agriculture's "Label Rouge" for products meeting stringent quality standards
Private standards referenced in regulation—Standards developed by the private sector that governments then reference	Private body—commercial or non-commercial	Legislation or regulatory agency	Private firms	Private or government auditor	Criminal or administrative courts	The U.S. Food Safety Modernization Act references approved third-party certifications
Voluntary private standards—Standards developed and adopted by private bodies. Often business-to-business standards	Private body—commercial or non-commercial	Private firms or organizations	Private firms	Private auditor	Private certification body	British Retail Consortium standards

SOURCES: Adapted from Garcia Martinez et al., 2013; Henson and Humphrey, 2010.

The use of third-party standards for food safety regulation is relatively common, partly because enforcement of food safety laws can be challenging given international supply chains (ACUS, 2012; Garcia Martinez et al., 2007). On one hand, compliance with third-party standards can help producers in low- and middle-income be competitive in more lucrative markets (Henson and Humphrey, 2010). At the same time, such standards are exacting and may block small farmers from market entry, though the evidence supporting such exclusion is mixed (Faour-Klingbeil and Todd, 2018; Henson and Humphrey, 2010).

Voluntary standards can be valuable tools for food suppliers looking to expand market access. Proof of animal welfare or environmental measures, as the Label Rouge certification referenced in Table 5-1 provides, can command a premium in certain market segments (Synalaf, 2013). Such standards should serve as a complement to, not as a substitute for, the core food safety protections regulatory agencies provide.

When viewed as a way to save on enforcement costs and increase the acceptability of regulatory policies, co-regulation can be a useful strategy for food regulators (Garcia Martinez et al., 2013). Because it involves a shift of emphasis from more reactive methods of regulation to prevention, it can also be appealing as a way to triage public resources (Rouvière and Caswell, 2012). Especially in food safety, the preventive approach, and one that makes good use of the wealth of information in internal inspections and process audits, is increasingly favored (Lin, 2014; Rouvière and Caswell, 2012). Perhaps for these reasons, voluntary certification schemes are gaining popularity in low- and middle-income countries (Jaffee et al., 2019). It may be too early to know how well these tools are working, but support from regulators, in the form of consumer education or endorsement of scientific certification schemes for example, could help these tools realize their maximum value (Jaffee et al., 2019). As FAO guidance on voluntary standards explained, the public sector has a responsibility to coordinate these standards so that they stimulate a market for safe foods, rather than serve as a barrier to entry, especially for small producers (UNEP and FAO, 2014).

As with regulatory cooperation, countries can share the infrastructure that supports quality. The Southern Africa Development Community, for example, has a regional accreditation body (SADCAS, n.d.-a). Established by the WTO's Technical Barriers to Trade Agreement, the program aims to improve laboratory services including testing, calibration, and medical laboratories in the region (Mutasa, 2014; SADCAS, n.d.-b). Accreditation from the regional authority provides an assurance of technical competence that many participating countries would not otherwise have, and it advances longer-term shared goals of protecting health and facilitating trade (Mutasa, 2014; SADCAS, n.d.-b).

The private sector also has an accreditation infrastructure in place that can enrich national training and compliance activities. At the same time, the private sector does not have the same motivators as government, and its prominence in regulation is controversial, seen to increase the already sizable power of large firms in the food market (ACUS, 2012; Garcia Martinez et al., 2007, 2013). For these reasons, co-regulation may work better in places where sophisticated understanding of regulatory goals is common in private firms (Garcia Martinez et al., 2013). To serve the goal of maximizing the value of staff time and resources, regulators should look for ways to make use of other organizations' work. Without wishing to set up a false equivalence between the resources available through UN agencies and those of the private sector, the committee encourages regulators to consider both as a starting point for establishing standards and monitoring quality.

Recommendation 5-3: National regulatory authorities should take advantage of global tools to support regulatory actions. Resources from United Nations agencies, including World Health Organization prequalification and Codex standards, are examples of such tools, as are the third-party standards increasingly used in food and agriculture.

Given the inevitable shortage of resources and the complicated, international nature of food and medicines production, there is an onus on the regulatory authority to seek the most efficient way to ensure product quality. There is valuable, credible information in third-party certification programs, as there is in the WHO prequalification assessment. Regulators can make use of these tools, as well as the publicly available Codex standards and guidelines in their work. An efficient use of such information can allow agencies in low- and middle-income countries more time and resources to combat risks unique to their contexts.

The committee recognizes that there is room for misuse or misunderstanding in implementing this recommendation. Even the relatively straightforward WHO prequalification program could be misused if regulators understood prequalification of one product as a transferable imprimatur to a manufacturer's entire product line. Particularly in its application to food safety, the potential for third-party tools to advantage larger businesses should be considered. The Administrative Conference of the United States recommends that, before deciding to use a third-party program to assess compliance, governments assess the capacity of the agency and the relative costs of the program, as well as the extent to which such programs may be unfair to small businesses. It encourages the regulatory agency to oversee third-party programs to ensure that they continue to advance the government's goals (as opposed to the market expansion goals of large companies) (ACUS, 2012).

Since third-party standards vary widely, it is difficult to comment on their likelihood of helping or harming small- and medium-sized producers in developing countries; research on such effects is mixed (Henson and Humphrey, 2010). The inclusion of experts from low- and middle-income countries on the governing boards and technical committees of standard-setting organizations, since they are in the Codex committees and the private Global GAP, is one strategy thought to promote inclusion (Henson and Humphrey, 2010).

This strategy also has implications for the way regulators approach their work. Most agencies, especially those in low- or middle-income countries, need good generalists, regulators with broad knowledge of the field who can make use of and judge the credibility of a range of technical documents (e.g., inspection reports, public assessments, and international guidelines such as those produced by Codex or the ICH). Small countries in particular rely on critical assessments of information produced abroad (Fefer, 2012). For example, Figure 5-2 shows how reliance might work for medicines registration, referencing the use of publicly available data from other agencies and the ICH Common Technical Document. The breadth of knowledge required makes the work challenging, and also unlike that of regulators in Europe or North America. Training and credentialing programs should reflect this distinction, and might be an area for the proposed Centers of Excellence in Regulatory Science to explore.

Efficiency and Delegating

The purpose of collaboration, co-regulation, and work sharing is to increase countries' efficiency, as well as to reduce restrictions on the movement of food and medicines internationally. Sparing resources allows agencies to attend to key local activities that others cannot perform, such as local inspections and controls on high-risk products sold in informal markets. But realizing the benefits of work sharing requires consideration of the full range of work sharing options, identifying those tasks that are best shared among different national governments and those that can be devolved to lower levels of government. In short, core policy work of the agency cannot be devolved to municipal or provincial authorities, though jobs may be delegated to the national agency that retains ultimate authority.

The risk-based framework described earlier in this report can be used to guide countries in identifying tasks suitable for the national agency, those better delegated to state or local authorities, and those candidates for international sharing. For example, a country may have data that allow the ranking of food safety risks based on disability-adjusted life years, or, as is more likely the case in low- and middle-income countries, it may rely on aggregate regional data on the same risks. New medicines approval may

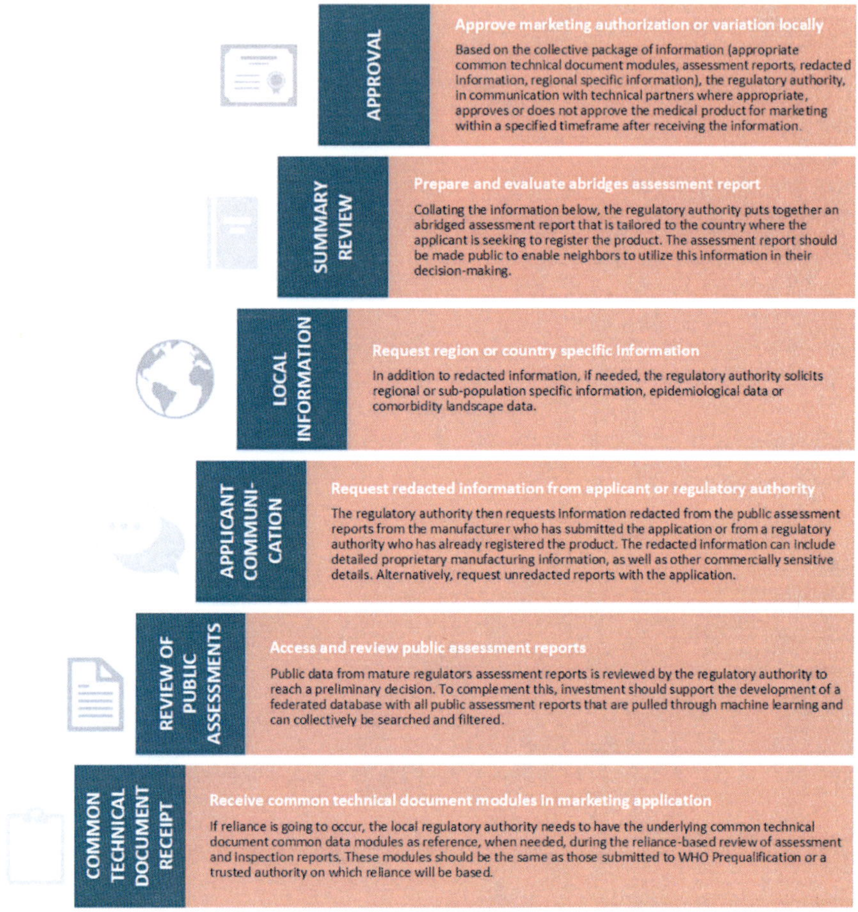
APPROVAL
Approve marketing authorization or variation locally
Based on the collective package of information (appropriate common technical document modules, assessment reports, redacted information, regional specific information), the regulatory authority, in communication with technical partners where appropriate, approves or does not approve the medical product for marketing within a specified timeframe after receiving the information.
SUMMARY REVIEW
Prepare and evaluate abridges assessment report
Collating the information below, the regulatory authority puts together an abridged assessment report that is tailored to the country where the applicant is seeking to register the product. The assessment report should be made public to enable neighbors to utilize this information in their decision-making.
LOCAL INFORMATION
Request region or country specific information
In addition to redacted information, if needed, the regulatory authority solicits regional or sub-population specific information, epidemiological data or comorbidity landscape data.
APPLICANT COMMUNI-CATION
Request redacted information from applicant or regulatory authority
The regulatory authority then requests information redacted from the public assessment reports from the manufacturer who has submitted the application or from a regulatory authority who has already registered the product. The redacted information can include detailed proprietary manufacturing information, as well as other commercially sensitive details. Alternatively, request unredacted reports with the application.
REVIEW OF PUBLIC ASSESSMENTS
Access and review public assessment reports
Public data from mature regulators assessment reports is reviewed by the regulatory authority to reach a preliminary decision. To complement this, investment should support the development of a federated database with all public assessment reports that are pulled through machine learning and can collectively be searched and filtered.
COMMON TECHNICAL DOCUMENT RECEIPT
Receive common technical document modules in marketing application
If reliance is going to occur, the local regulatory authority needs to have the underlying common technical document common data modules as reference, when needed, during the reliance-based review of assessment and inspection reports. These modules should be the same as those submitted to WHO Prequalification or a trusted authority on which reliance will be based.

FIGURE 5-2 Steps to implement reliance for medicines registration.
SOURCE: Roth et al., 2018.

rely on a country's own review, a joint review with neighboring countries, or the acceptance of a trusted foreign authority's review.

The idea of a regulatory value chain can also be useful in organizing work sharing and delegation (Chahal et al., 2016). Figure 5-3 shows core regulatory activities in the top band; those further to the left are candidates for regional regulatory cooperation or the unilateral acceptance of a trusted authority's work. Those post-market tasks on the right of the band, including communication with the public, testing, and issuing recalls, are essentially domestic jobs, with some elements of them ripe for delegation to provincial or municipal authorities.

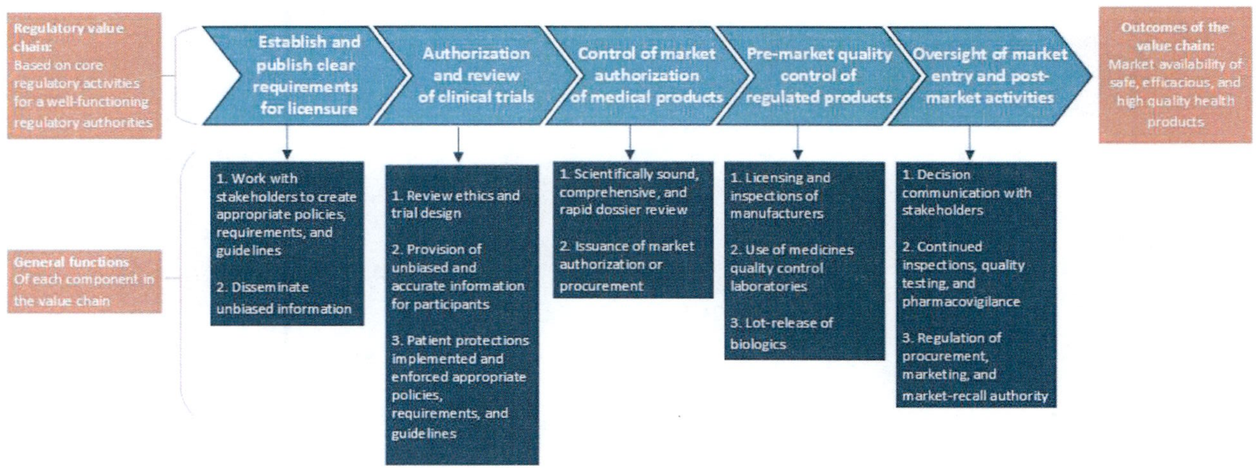

FIGURE 5-3 A regulatory value chain for medicines regulation.
SOURCE: Adapted from Chahal et al., 2016.

Regulatory agencies often work at multiple levels of government (Jaffee et al., 2019; Kaddu et al., 2018). There is no universal blueprint for making the public sector more efficient, but communication among government agencies, both at the level of the national government and at various subnational levels, will always be crucial (Curristine et al., 2007). In terms of managing food and medicines, there are tasks such as the inspection of pharmacies and restaurants that lend themselves to oversight at provincial or municipal levels. When more than one level of government is responsible for advancing larger policy objectives, considerable coordination among those levels becomes important (Charbit and Muichalun, 2009).

A 2009 analysis for the OECD found "duplication of rules, overlapping and low-quality regulations, and uneven enforcement" to be the most common problems when sharing regulatory responsibilities at different levels of government (Charbit and Muichalun, 2009). Capacity is often not as strong at sub-national levels, especially for technical work (Smoke, 2015). Partly because of financial limitations, it is difficult for subnational levels of government to maintain the staff or other resources, such as laboratories (Charbit and Muichalun, 2009).

Research in Malawi found the food inspection services at the district and city levels to be severely understaffed and noted confusion regarding guidelines, standards, and enforcement, problems only complicated by the variety of ministries with food safety responsibilities (e.g., agriculture, tourism, health) (Morse et al., 2018). It may stand to reason that in countries with a more federal system of government, the pathway for delegation would be more clear, but it is not necessarily so. Medicines regulation in India, for example, is shared between the central and state governments (Gupta et al., 2017). The state authorities have sole responsibility for distribution and sale, as well as most of the authority for licensing and inspecting manufacturers (exceptions are made for high-risk products, WHO manufacturing inspections, and certain federal jurisdictions) (Chowdhury et al., 2015). In practice, regulatory implementation varies widely among states (Chowdhury et al., 2015; Ministry of Health and Family Welfare, 2003). In some places, licensing works well, but others have problems (Chowdhury et al., 2015). Managing the uneven quality of the state authorities is a significant challenge for the national agency.

Inspectors may fear for their safety in places were unscrupulous manufacturers have ties to organized crime; the inspectors' obligation to appear in court can compound the problem and takes time away from inspecting (Chowdhury et al., 2015). Quality testing is also problematic; in some states in India central testing labs lack the equipment for the full range of assays (Chowdhury et al., 2015). In India, as in much of the world, there can be an emphasis on putting the national system in place, forgetting that a lot of the pieces depend on effective work at sub-national levels (Morse et al., 2018).

Recommendation 5-4: National regulatory authorities should determine which functions are most effectively and efficiently carried out directly by the agency and which can be delegated to state or local authorities; collaboration and data sharing among domestic agencies should be part of any delegation plan.

Analyses of devolution programs in low- and middle-income countries have found that when decentralization happens quickly, there may be confusion over roles and conflict among staff (Cobos Munoz et al., 2017; Nxumalo et al., 2018). Sufficient funding for the increased burden on district and local offices is important, as is taking time to train staff for their new roles (Nxumalo et al., 2018). Fostering good relationships across levels and coordinating policies to avoid overlap or conflicting roles should be a priority in any delegation or devolution plan (Charbit and Muichalun, 2009).

One of the main challenges of cooperating across levels of government is in information sharing. Local offices may have extensive information on small parts of a problem, but this information needs to be shared and managed across levels (Charbit and Muichalun, 2009). Furthermore, the availability of technology at subnational levels of government is less likely in low- and middle-income countries, making even data collection more difficult (Brack and Castillo, 2015). Technological limitations, while challenging, can be an opportunity. Chatham House recommends putting the basic foundation for data literacy in place before implementing a data policy that may be unsuitable to the local context (Brack and Castillo, 2015). Especially in places where data sharing is new, it is also important to articulate a clear and compelling argument for data sharing, framing it in terms of the benefits accrued to society at large and to individual stakeholders (Brack and Castillo, 2015).

Another common obstacle to work sharing is having sufficient funding for all jobs delegated to provincial or municipal authorities (Cobos Munoz et al., 2017). The central government always has an advantage in collecting revenue (Smoke, 2015). When sub-national governments do not have reliable income, transfer from the federal government might be necessary (Charbit and Muichalun, 2009). There are also strategies the national government can take on to pool resources and help subnational levels build economies of scale (Charbit and Muichalun, 2009). The Food Emergency Response Network, for example, gives various state, local, and tribal food safety laboratories protected surge capacity during large-scale outbreaks (FDA, 2018a). During an emergency, the national network coordinator schedules increased testing across various network laboratories, speeding response time; the program also supports some sites to develop new analytic methods (FDA, 2018a; ICLN, n.d.).

Delegation and work sharing also require capacity building, both in increasing technical capacity, mostly at the lower levels, and in increasing governance capacity—meaning developing the skills and protocols that allow the levels to work together—at all levels (Smoke, 2015). Clarity in the division of work can go far to improving cooperation (Curristine et al., 2007; Smoke, 2015). Programs that build networks and bring regulators from different levels together can also improve governance capacity, creating a mutually reinforcing cycle of cooperation and capacity building (Charbit and Muichalun, 2009).

There is a mutual dependence among levels of government. In delegating or sharing work among those levels it is important to be clear about who answers to whom and that everyone answers to someone (Nxumalo et al., 2018). District and local regulators may feel greater accountability to local authorities, but even in highly decentralized systems, there is usually also some degree of accountability to the central government; balancing the priorities and accountability among these levels can be challenging (Nxumalo et al., 2018). Some evidene suggests that good professional relationships among staff at different levels can build accountability, causing people to feel that they are all on the same team (Nxumalo et al., 2018).

The national regulatory authority has a responsibility to set the subnational offices up for success, taking stock of the risks facing the country and setting priorities accordingly. In India, for example, where medicines manufacturing is the main driver of the market, inspection against good manufacturing practices will take precedence (Chowdhury et al., 2015). The national government may also need to give grants to states to help them upgrade their facilities (Chowdhury et al., 2015).

REFERENCES

Abrahams, C. 2009. Transforming the region: Supermarkets and the local food economy. *African Affairs* 109(434):115–134.

Access to Medicine Foundation. 2018. *Access to medicines index 2018*. Amsterdam, Netherlands: Access to Medicine Foundation.

ACUS (Administrative Conference of the United States). 2012. *Administrative conference recommendation 2012–7: Agency use of third-party programs to assess regulatory compliance*. https://www.acus.gov/sites/default/files/documents/Recommendation%20 2012-7%20%28Third-Party%20Programs%20to%20Assess%20Regulatory%20Compliance%29.pdf (accessed August 29, 2019).

Ahonkhai, V., S. F. Martins, A. Portet, M. Lumpkin, and D. Hartman. 2016. Speeding access to vaccines and medicines in low- and middle-income countries: A case for change and a framework for optimized product market authorization. *PLoS One* 11(11):e0166515.

Alcorn, T., and Y. Ouyang. 2012. China's invisible burden of foodborne illness. *The Lancet* 379(9818):789–790.

Aminu, N., A. Sha'aban, A. Abubakar, and M. S. Gwarzo. 2017. Unveiling the peril of substandard and falsified medicines to public health and safety in Africa: Need for all-out war to end the menace. *Medicine Access @ Point of Care* 1:maapoc.0000023.

Anderson, R. 2011. Apple juice is still safe, FDA says. Food Safety News. https://www.foodsafetynews.com/2011/11/apple-juice-is-still-safe-fda-insists (accessed August 20, 2019).

Andrews, J. 2012. 2009 Peanut butter outbreak: Three years on, still no resolution for some. Food Safety News. https://www.foodsafetynews.com/2012/04/2009-peanut-butter-outbreak-three-years-on-still-no-resolution-for-some (accessed August 20, 2019).

APEC (Asia-Pacific Economic Cooperation). 2018. *APEC food safety capacity building initiative: Update to the mid-term review*. http://fscf-ptin.apec.org/docs/2018/2018_Independent_Review_of_APEC_FSCF_PTIN_Food_Safety_Capacity_Building_Report.pdf (accessed August 20, 2019).

Arriola Penalosa, M. A., R. Cavazos Cepeda, M. Alanis Garza, and M. M. Lumpkin. 2017. Optimized medical product regulation in Mexico: A win-win for public and economic health. *Therapeutic Innovation & Regulatory Science* 51(6):744–750.

Babigumira, J. B., A. Stergachis, T. Kanyok, L. Evans, M. Hajjou, P. O. Nkansah, V. Pribluda, J. Louis P. Garrison, and J. I. Nwokike. 2018. *A risk-based resource allocation framework for pharmaceutical quality assurance for medicines regulatory authorities in low- and middle-income countries*. Rockville, MD: USAID.

Baldwin, R. 2014. From regulation to behaviour change: Giving nudge the third degree. *The Modern Law Review* 77(6):831–857.

Bezuidenhout, L., and E. Chakauya. 2018. Hidden concerns of sharing research data by low/middle-income country scientists. *Global bioethics = Problemi di bioetica* 29(1):39–54.

Bloom, G., S. Henson, and D. H. Peters. 2014. Innovation in regulation of rapidly changing health markets. *Global Health* 10(1):53.

Bloomberg News. 2019. *China's lethal milk scandal reverberates a decade later.* https://www.bloomberg.com/news/articles/2019-01-21/china-s-lethal-milk-scandal-reverberates-a-decade-later (accessed August 20, 2019).

Boin, A., P. 't. Hart, E. Stern, and B. Sundelius. 2005. *The politics of crisis: Public leadership under pressure*. Cambridge, UK: Cambridge University Press.

Brack, M., and T. Castillo. 2015. *Data sharing for public health: Key lessons from other sectors*. London, UK: Chatham House, The Royal Institute for International Affairs. https://www.chathamhouse.org/publication/data-sharing-public-health-key-lessons-other-sectors (accessed December 8, 2019).

Bresnick, J. 2019. *Is healthcare any closer to achieving the promises of big data analytics?* https://healthitanalytics.com/news/is-healthcare-any-closer-to-achieving-the-promises-of-big-data-analytics (accessed August 16, 2019).

Browne, D. 2018. Fixing a crisis of confidence in drug compounding. *Washington Examiner.* https://www.washingtonexaminer.com/fixing-a-crisis-of-confidence-in-drug-compounding (accessed February 13, 2020).

Caipo, M. 2019. *FAO/WHO Food Control System Assessment Tool*. Paper presented to Committee on Stronger Food and Drug Regulatory Systems Abroad, February 25, San Jose, Costa Rica.

Cancer Research UK. 2019. *Phases of clinical trials*. https://www.cancerresearchuk.org/about-cancer/find-a-clinical-trial/what-clinical-trials-are/phases-of-clinical-trials#phase4 (accessed August 28, 2019).

CDC (U.S. Centers for Disease Control and Prevention). 2010. *Multistate outbreak of human* Salmonella enteritidis *infections associated with shell eggs (Final update)*. https://www.cdc.gov/salmonella/2010/shell-eggs-12-2-10.html (accessed August 20, 2019).

CDC. 2014. *CERC manual*. https://emergency.cdc.gov/cerc/manual/index.asp (accessed August 20, 2019).

Chahal, H. S., F. Kashfipour, M. Susko, N. S. Feachem, and C. Boyle. 2016. Establishing a regulatory value chain model: An innovative approach to strengthening medicines regulatory systems in resource-constrained settings. *Revista Panamericana de Salud Pública* 39(5):299–305.

Chakraborty, S., and R. Lofstedt. 2012. Transparency initiative by the FDA's Center for Drug Evaluation and Research (CDER): Two qualitative studies of public perceptions. *European Journal of Risk Regulation* 3(1):57–71.

Chalker, J. C., C. Vialle-Valentin, J. Liana, R. Mbwasi, I. A. Semali, B. Kihiyo, E. Shekalaghe, A. Dillip, S. Kimatta, R. Valimba, M. Embrey, R. Lieber, E. Rutta, K. Johnson, and D. Ross-Degnan. 2015. What roles do accredited drug dispensing outlets in Tanzania play in facilitating access to antimicrobials? Results of a multi-method analysis. *Antimicrobial Resistance and Infection Control* 4(1):33.

Charbit, C., and M. Muichalun. 2009. Mind the gaps: Managing mutual dependence in relations among levels of government. OECD Working Papers on Public Governance No. 14. Paris, France: OECD.

Cheah, P. Y. 2019. Institutions must state policy on data sharing. *Nature International Journal of Science* 565.

Chinwendu, O. 2008. *The fight against fake drugs by NAFDAC in Nigeria*. Paper presented at 44th International Course in Health Development (ICHD), September 24, 2007–September 12, 2008, Amsterdam, Netherlands.

Chowdhury, N., P. Joshi, A. Patnaik, and B. Saraswathy. 2015. *Administrative structure and functions of drug regulatory authorities in India*. Working paper. New Delhi, India: Indian Council for Research on International Economic Relations.

Cobos Munoz, D., P. Merino Amador, L. Monzon Llamas, D. Martinez Hernandez, and J. M. Santos Sancho. 2017. Decentralization of health systems in low and middle income countries: A systematic review. *International Journal of Public Health* 62(2):219–229.

Cooper, L. V., A. Robson, C. L. Trotter, A. Aseffa, J. M. Collard, D. M. Daugla, A. Diallo, A. Hodgson, J. F. Jusot, B. Omotara, S. Sow, M. Hassan-King, O. Manigart, M. Nascimento, A. Woukeu, D. Chandramohan, R. Borrow, M. C. J. Maiden, B. Greenwood, J. M. Stuart, and C. MenAfriCar. 2019. Risk factors for acquisition of meningococcal carriage in the African meningitis belt. *Tropical Medicine & International Health* 24(4):392–400.

Curristine, T., Z. Lonti, and I. Joumard. 2007. Improving public sector efficiency. *OECD Journal on Budgeting* 7(1):1–41.

Daugla, D. M., J. P. Gami, K. Gamougam, N. Naibei, L. Mbainadji, M. Narbe, J. Toralta, B. Kodbesse, C. Ngadoua, M. E. Coldiron, F. Fermon, A. L. Page, M. H. Djingarey, S. Hugonnet, O. B. Harrison, L. S. Rebbetts, Y. Tekletsion, E. R. Watkins, D. Hill, D. A. Caugant, D. Chandramohan, M. Hassan-King, O. Manigart, M. Nascimento, A. Woukeu, C. Trotter, J. M. Stuart, M. Maiden, and B. M. Greenwood. 2014. Effect of a serogroup A meningococcal conjugate vaccine (PSA-TT) on serogroup A meningococcal meningitis and carriage in Chad: A community study [corrected]. *The Lancet* 383(9911):40–47.

De Groote, H., C. Narrod, S. C. Kimenju, C. Bett, R. P. B. Scott, M. M. Tiongco, and Z. M. Gitonga. 2016. Measuring rural consumers' willingness to pay for quality labels using experimental auctions: The case of aflatoxin-free maize in Kenya. *Agricultural Economics* 47(1):33–45.

Dulli, L. 2019. Mobile technology for sexual and reproductive health interventions in low- and middle-income countries. *American Journal of Public Health* 109(6):836–837.

EDCTP (European and Developing Countries Clinical Trials Partnership). n.d. *Home*. http://www.edctp.org (accessed October 22, 2019).

EDCTP Knowledge Hub. n.d.-a. *Data sharing toolkit*. https://edctpknowledgehub.tghn.org/data-sharing-toolkit (accessed October 22, 2019).

EDCTP Knowledge Hub. n.d.-b. *Home*. https://edctpknowledgehub.tghn.org (accessed October 22, 2019).

El-Jardali, F., E. A. Akl, R. Fadlallah, S. Oliver, N. Saleh, L. El-Bawab, R. Rizk, A. Farha, and R. Hamra. 2015. Interventions to combat or prevent drug counterfeiting: A systematic review. *BMJ Open* 5(3):e006290.

Embrey, M., C. Vialle-Valentin, A. Dillip, B. Kihiyo, R. Mbwasi, I. A. Semali, J. C. Chalker, J. Liana, R. Lieber, K. Johnson, E. Rutta, S. Kimatta, E. Shekalaghe, R. Valimba, and D. Ross-Degnan. 2016. Understanding the role of accredited drug dispensing outlets in Tanzania's health system. *PLoS One* 11(11):e0164332.

FAO (Food and Agriculture Organization of the United Nations). 2016. *Influencing food environments for healthy diets*. Rome, Italy: FAO.

FAO and WHO (World Health Organization). 2016. *Risk communication applied to food safety handbook*. Rome, Italy: FAO.

FAO, WHO, and WTO (World Trade Organization). 2019. *Joint statement by FAO, WHO, and WTO: International forum on food safety and trade (23–24 April 2019, Geneva, Switzerland)*. https://www.who.int/docs/default-source/resources/joint-statement.pdf?sfvrsn=61b890c4_2 (accessed August 21, 2019).

Faour-Klingbeil, D., and E. C. D. Todd. 2018. A review on the rising prevalence of international standards: Threats or opportunities for the agri-food produce sector in developing countries, with a focus on examples from the mena region. *Foods* 7(3).

Fatokun, O. 2016. Curbing the circulation of counterfeit medicines in Nigeria. *The Lancet* 388(10060):2603.

FDA (U.S. Food and Drug Administration). 2008. In *Get notified about the U.S. Food and Drug Administration's recalls. Privacy Policy.* @FDArecalls: Twitter. http://www.fda.gov/privacy (accessed February 13, 2019).

FDA. 2018a. *Food emergency response network (FERN)*. https://www.fda.gov/federal-state-local-tribal-and-territorial-officials/grants-and-cooperative-agreements/food-emergency-response-network-fern (accessed September 18, 2019).

FDA. 2018b. *Frances Oldham Kelsey: Medical reviewer famous for averting a public health tragedy*. https://www.fda.gov/about-fda/virtual-exhibits-fda-history/frances-oldham-kelsey-medical-reviewer-famous-averting-public-health-tragedy (accessed August 21, 2019).

FDA. 2019. *Economic impact analyses of FDA regulations*. https://www.fda.gov/about-fda/reports/economic-impact-analyses-fda-regulations (accessed August 20, 2019).

FDA. n.d. *FDA's risk communication research agenda*. https://www.fda.gov/media/79104/download (accessed August 20, 2019).

Fefer, E. 2012. Pharmaceutical legislation and regulation. In *MDS-3: Managing access to medicines and health technologies*. Arlington, VA: Management Sciences for Health.

Fontannaz-Aujoulat, F., M. Frost, and J. Schlundt. 2019. WHO five keys to safer food communication campaign—Evidence-based simple messages with a global impact. *Food Control* 101:53–57.

FSSAI (Food Safety and Standards Authority of India). n.d. *Success stories*. https://snfportal.in/snf/jsp/csf_success.jsp (accessed August 20, 2019).

Fuhr, T., K. George, and J. Pai. 2013. *The business case for medical device quality.* McKinsey Center for Government. https://docplayer.net/8550902-Mckinsey-center-for-government-the-business-case-for-medical-device-quality.html (accessed December 8, 2019).

Garcia Martinez, M., A. Fearne, J. A. Caswell, and S. Henson. 2007. Co-regulation as a possible model for food safety governance: Opportunities for public–private partnerships. *Food Policy* 32(3):299–314.

Garcia Martinez, M., P. Verbruggen, and A. Fearne. 2013. Risk-based approaches to food safety regulation: What role for co-regulation? *Journal of Risk Research* 16(9):1101–1121.

Garg, V., S. Chopra, S. Singh, M. Gulati, B. Kumar, and N. Mittal Garg. 2017. A comparative study of common technical document in different regulated market. *Journal of Pharmacy Research* 11:1015–1024.

GFSP (Global Food Safety Partnership). n.d. *About UA*. https://www.gfsp.org/about-us (accessed October 7, 2019).

Goodman, C., W. Brieger, A. Unwin, A. Mills, S. Meek, and G. Greer. 2007. Medicine sellers and malaria treatment in sub-Saharan Africa: What do they do and how can their practice be improved? *American Journal of Tropical Medicine and Hygiene* 77(6 Suppl):203–218.

Gostin, L. O. 2018. *Public health law and ethics: A reader*. 3rd ed. Berkeley and Los Angeles, CA: University of California Press.

Grace, D. 2015a. Food safety in low and middle income countries. *International Journal of Environmental Research and Public Health* 12(9):10490–10507.

Grace, D. 2015b. Taking food safety to informal markets. In *Food safety and informal markets: Animal products in Sub-Saharan Africa*, edited by K. Roesel and D. Grace. Oxford, UK: Taylor & Francis Group.

Grace, D., K. Roesel, and T. Lore. 2014. *Food safety in informal markets in developing countries: Lessons from research by the International Livestock Research Institute*. https://pdfs.semanticscholar.org/d41b/923fef6d4b0207c36698123483f16b8c5196.pdf (accessed September 6, 2019).

Grace, D., M. Dipeolu, and S. Alonso. 2019. Improving food safety in the informal sector: Nine years later. *Infection Ecology & Epidemiology* 9(1):1579613.

Greenemeier, L. 2008. Heparin scare: Deaths from tainted blood-thinner spur race for safe replacement. *Scientific American*. https://www.scientificamerican.com/article/heparin-scare-deaths (accessed August 20, 2019).

Gupta, M., M. Shridhar, G. N. Singh, and A. Khadem. 2017. Regulatory systems in India: An important global hub for medical products and technologies. *WHO Drug Information* 31(3).

Hajduk, G. K., N. E. Jamieson, B. L. Baker, O. F. Olesen, and T. Lang. 2019. It is not enough that we require data to be shared; we have to make sharing easy, feasible and accessible too! *BMJ Global Health* 4(4):e001550.

Halabi, S. F., and C. F. Lin. 2017. Assessing the relative influence and efficacy of public and private food safety regulation regimes: Comparing Codex and global GAP standards. *Food and Drug Law Journal* 72(2):262–294.

Hamilton, W. L., C. Doyle, M. Halliwell-Ewen, and G. Lambert. 2016. Public health interventions to protect against falsified medicines: A systematic review of international, national and local policies. *Health Policy and Planning* 31(10):1448–1466.

Harkins, M. W. 2016. External partnerships: The power of sharing information. In *Managing risk and information security*, edited by M. W. Harkins. Berkeley, CA: Apress. Pp. 49–63.

Harris, G. 2006. F.D.A. Warns against eating bag spinach. *The New York Times*. https://www.nytimes.com/2006/09/15/us/15spinach.html (accessed December 8, 2019).

Henson, S., and J. Humphrey. 2010. Understanding the complexities of private standards in global agri-food chains as they impact developing countries. *Journal of Development Studies* 46(9):1628–1646.

Hermann, C. F. 1969. *Crises in foreign policy: A simulation analysis (advanced study in political science)*. Indianapolis, IN: Bobbs-Merrill.

HHS (U.S. Department of Health and Human Services). n.d. *HIV/AIDS glossary: Phase 4 trial*. https://aidsinfo.nih.gov/understanding-hiv-aids/glossary/571/phase-4-trial (accessed December 8, 2019).

Hogerzeil, H. V., J. K. Iyer, L. Urlings, T. Prasad, and S. Brewer. 2014. Is the pharmaceutical industry improving with regard to access to essential medicines? *The Lancet Global Health* 2(3):e139–e140.

IBM (International Business Machines) Corporation. 2019. *About IBM food trust.* https://www.ibm.com/downloads/cas/8QABQBDR (accessed August 20, 2019).

ICH (International Council for Harmonisation of Technical Requirements for Pharmaceuticals for Human Use). n.d. *M4: The common technical document.* https://www.ich.org/products/ctd.html (accessed August 27, 2019).

ICLN (Integrated Consortium of Laboratory Networks). n.d. *FERN.* https://www.icln.org/fern (accessed September 18, 2019).

ILRI (International Livestock Research Institute). 2010a. Assessing consumer preferences for quality and safety attributes of food in the absence of official standards: The case of beef, raw milk and local butter in Ethiopia. In *Demand for livestock products in developing countries with a focus on quality and safety attributes: Evidence from case studies*, edited by M. A. Jabbar, D. Baker, and M. L. Fadiga. Nairobi, Kenya, and Addis Ababa, Ethiopia: International Livestock Research Institute.

ILRI. 2010b. *Demand for livestock products in developing countries with a focus on quality and safety attributes: Evidence from case studies.* Nairobi, Kenya, and Addis Ababa, Ethiopia: International Livestock Research Institute.

ILRI. 2010c. Introduction. In *Demand for livestock products in developing countries with a focus on quality and safety attributes: Evidence from case studies*, edited by M. A. Jabbar, D. Baker, and M. L. Fadiga. Nairobi, Kenya, and Addis Ababa, Ethiopia: International Livestock Research Institute.

ILRI. n.d. *Food safety in informal markets.* https://safefoodfairfood.ilri.org/food-safety-in-informal-markets (accessed September 6, 2019).

Instituto Nacional de Salud Pública de México. 2016. *Review of current labelling regulations and practices for food and beverage targeting children and adolescents in Latin America countries (Mexico, Chile, Costa Rica and Argentina) and recommendations for facilitating consumer information.* New York: UNICEF.

IOM (Institute of Medicine). 2012. *Ensuring safe foods and medical products through stronger regulatory systems abroad.* Washington, DC: The National Academies Press.

IOM. 2013. *Countering the problem of falsified and substandard drugs.* Washington, DC: The National Academies Press.

IOM and NRC (National Research Council). 2010a. Adopting a risk-based decision-making approach to food safety. In *Enhancing food safety: The role of the Food and Drug Administration.* Washington, DC: The National Academies Press. P. 588.

IOM and NRC. 2010b. *Enhancing food safety: The role of the Food and Drug Administration.* Washington, DC: The National Academies Press.

Jaffee, S., S. Henson, L. Unnevehr, D. Grace, and E. Cassou. 2019. *The safe food imperative : Accelerating progress in low- and middle-income countries.* Agriculture and food series. Washington, DC: World Bank.

Jessup, A. 2013. *Cost-benefit analysis at HHS.* http://nationalacademies.org/hmd/~/media/Files/Activity%20Files/Nutrition/AssessingFoodSystems/Sept%20Workshop/Presentations/Jessup%20NAS%20presentation%209-17-13.pdf (accessed August 20, 2019).

Kaale, E., V. Manyanga, M. Chambuso, J. Liana, E. Rutta, M. Embrey, T. Layloff, and K. Johnson. 2016. The quality of selected essential medicines sold in accredited drug dispensing outlets and pharmacies in Tanzania. *PLoS One* 11(11):e0165785.

Kaddu, G., E. D'Amore, A. Clark, and P. Nkansah. 2018. *Strengthening regulatory systems to improve medical product quality in low- and middle-income countries.* Rockville, MD: Promoting the Quality of Medicines (PQM) program. U.S. Pharmacopeial Convention.

Knowledge@Wharton. 2018. *How the blockchain brings social benefits to emerging economies.* https://knowledge.wharton.upenn.edu/article/blockchain-brings-social-benefits-emerging-economies (accessed August 20, 2019).

Lapar, L., and N. Toan. 2010. *Demand for pork by Vietnamese consumers: Implications for pro-poor livestock policy and development agenda in Vietnam.* Nairobi, Kenya: ILRI.

Larson, H. J. 2018. The biggest pandemic risk? Viral misinformation. *Nature* 562(7727):309.

Lau, A. Y., E. Gabarron, L. Fernandez-Luque, and M. Armayones. 2012. Social media in health—What are the safety concerns for health consumers? *Health Information Management Journal* 41(2):30–35.

Liana, J. H. 2014. *The Accredited Drug Dispensing Outlet (ADDO) model in Tanzania.* http://www.nationalacademies.org/hmd/~/media/Files/Activity%20Files/Research/NeuroForum/2014-JAN-13/22%20Liana%20presentation.pdf (accessed September 18, 2019).

Lin, C. F. 2014. Public–private interactions in global food safety governance. *Food and Drug Law Journal* 69(2):143–160.

Lu, Y., P. Hernandez, D. Abegunde, and T. Edejer. 2011. *The world medicines situation 2011: Medicine expenditures.* Geneva, Switzerland: WHO.

Luigetti, R., P. Bachmann, E. Cooke, and T. Salmonson. 2016. Collaboration, not competition: Developing new reliance models—regulatory collaboration. Exchange of assessment reports (ARS) with regulators outside the European Union (EU). *WHO Drug Information* 30(4):9.

Mackey, T. K., and G. Nayyar. 2017. A review of existing and emerging digital technologies to combat the global trade in fake medicines. *Expert Opinion on Drug Safety* 16(5):587–602.

Meserole, C. 2018. How misinformation spreads on social media—and what to do about it. Brookings. https://www.brookings.edu/blog/order-from-chaos/2018/05/09/how-misinformation-spreads-on-social-media-and-what-to-do-about-it (accessed August 20, 2019).

Ministry of Health and Family Welfare (Government of India). 2003. *Report of the expert committee on a comprehensive examination of drug regulatory issues, including the problem of spurious drugs.* http://planningcommission.nic.in/reports/genrep/health/Final_Report_mashelkar.pdf (accessed August 22, 2019).

Moon, S., J. A. Rottingen, and J. Frenk. 2017. Global public goods for health: Weaknesses and opportunities in the global health system. *Health Economics, Policy and Law* 12(2):195–205.

Morse, T. D., H. Masuku, S. Rippon, and H. Kubwalo. 2018. Achieving an integrated approach to food safety and hygiene—meeting the sustainable development goals in sub-Saharan Africa. *Sustainability* 10(7):2394.

MSH (Management Sciences for Health). 2013. *Providing access to medicines and health: A conversation with two women Accredited Drug Dispensing Outlet (ADDO) owners—Part 1: Meet Audensia.* https://www.msh.org/blog/2013/09/20/providing-access-to-medicines-and-health-a-conversation-with-two-women-accredited (accessed September 18, 2019).

Mutasa, M. P. 2014. *SADCAS experiences—Medical laboratories accreditation programme.* Paper read at MLAP-SLMTA/SLIPTA Symposium, November 28–29, 2014, Cape Town, South Africa.

NAFDAC (National Agency for Food and Drug Administration and Control). 2016. *NAFDAC good distribution practices guidelines for pharmaceutical products 2016.* Abuja, Nigeria: NAFDAC.

Narrod, C., X. Dao, M. Miller, and C. Wychgram. 2019a. Public private partnerships in food safety international capacity building. In *Food safety economics—Incentives for a safer food supply*, edited by T. Roberts. Cham, Switzerland: Springer Nature.

Narrod, C., A. Stumpf, and X. Dou. 2019b (unpublished). *Harnessing public–private partnerships for data sharing to measure the impact of food safety capacity building.*

NASEM (National Academies of Sciences, Engineering, and Medicine). 2018. *Crossing the global quality chasm: Improving health care worldwide*. Washington, DC: The National Academies Press.

Nxumalo, N., L. Gilson, J. Goudge, B. Tsofa, S. Cleary, E. Barasa, and S. Molyneux. 2018. Accountability mechanisms and the value of relationships: Experiences of front-line managers at subnational level in Kenya and South Africa. *British Medical Journal* 3(4).

OECD (Organisation for Economic Co-operation and Development). 2013. *International regulatory co-operation—Better rules of globalisation*. http://www.oecd.org/gov/regulatory-policy/irc.htm (accessed December 8, 2019).

OECD. 2016. Being an independent regulator. In *The Governance of Regulators*. Paris, France: OECD Publishing. https://www.oecd-ilibrary.org/content/publication/9789264209015-en (accessed August 9, 2019).

OECD. 2018. Assessment and recommendations. In *Review of international regulatory co-operation of Mexico*. Paris, France: OECD Publishing.

OECD. n.d.-a. *A MENA-OECD practitioners' guide for engaging stakeholders in the rule-making process*. https://www.oecd.org/mena/governance/MENA-Practitioners-Guide-%20EN.pdf (accessed August 20, 2019).

OECD. n.d.-b. *Regulatory impact analysis*. https://www.oecd.org/regreform/regulatory-policy/ria.htm (accessed August 20, 2019).

Office of Information and Regulatory Affairs. 2011. *Regulatory impact analysis: A primer*. Circular A-4. https://www.whitehouse.gov/sites/whitehouse.gov/files/omb/inforeg/inforeg/regpol/circular-a-4_regulatory-impact-analysis-a-primer.pdf (accessed October 7, 2019).

Ortega, D. L., and D. L. Tschirley. 2017. Demand for food safety in emerging and developing countries. *Journal of Agribusiness in Developing and Emerging Economies* 7(1):21–34.

Ostroff, S. 2018. The costs of foodborne illness, product recalls make the case for food safety investments. *Food Safety Magazine*. https://www.foodsafetymagazine.com/magazine-archive1/junejuly-2018/the-costs-of-foodborne-illness-product-recalls-make-the-case-for-food-safety-investments (accessed December 8, 2019).

Paoli, G. 2010. *Quantitative risk assessment analysis training material*. College Park, MD: University of Maryland, Joint Institute for Food Safety and Applied Nutrition.

Parker, D., and C. Kirkpatrick. 2012. *The economic impact of regulatory policy: A literature review of quantitative evidence*. Paris, France: OECD.

Perez-Escamilla, R., C. K. Lutter, C. Rabadan-Diehl, A. Rubinstein, A. Calvillo, C. Corvalan, C. Batis, E. Jacoby, S. Vorkoper, L. Kline, E. Ewart-Pierce, and J. A. Rivera. 2017. Prevention of childhood obesity and food policies in Latin America: From research to practice. *Obesity Reviews* 18 Suppl 2(S2):28–38.

PharmaSecure. n.d. *Nigeria—NAFDAS MAS*. https://www.pharmasecure.com/mas-nigeria (accessed November 14, 2019).

Pisa, M., and D. McCurdy. 2019. *Improving global health supply chains through traceability*. Washington, DC: Center for Global Development.

Pisani, E. 2019. How moves towards universal health coverage could encourage poor quality drugs: An essay by Elizabeth Pisani. *BMJ* 366:l5327.

Poole, K. E., and E. D. Harpel. 2018. *Advancing state data sharing for better economic and workforce development*. Arlington, VA: Center for Regional Economic Competitiveness.

Raghupathi, W., and V. Raghupathi. 2014. Big data analytics in healthcare: Promise and potential. *Health Information Science and Systems* 2:3.

Resnick, D. 2017. Governance: Informal food markets in Africa's cities. In *2017 Global food policy report*. Washington, DC: IFPRI.

Reuters. 2007. *U.S. Seizes tainted toothpaste from China.* https://www.reuters.com/article/us-toothpaste-fda/u-s-seizes-tainted-toothpaste-from-china-idUSWAT00764420070601 (accessed November 22, 2019).

Roesel, K., and D. Grace. 2014. *Food safety and informal markets: Animal products in sub-Saharan Africa.* London, UK: Routledge.

Roth, L., D. Bempong, J. B. Babigumira, S. Banoo, E. Cooke, D. Jeffreys, L. Kasonde, H. G. M. Leufkens, J. C. W. Lim, M. Lumpkin, G. Mahlangu, R. W. Peeling, H. Rees, M. Ndomondo-Sigonda, A. Stergachis, M. Ward, and J. Nwokike. 2018. Expanding global access to essential medicines: Investment priorities for sustainably strengthening medical product regulatory systems. *Global Health* 14(1):102.

Rouvière, E., and J. A. Caswell. 2012. From punishment to prevention: A French case study of the introduction of co-regulation in enforcing food safety. *Food Policy* 37(3):246–254.

Rutta, E. 2014. Chapter 5—Annex 1: Accredited drug dispensing outlets. In *Alliance for health policy and systems research flagship report 2014.* Geneva, Switzerland: WHO.

SADCAS (Southern Africa Development Community Accreditation Service). n.d.-a. *Home.* https://www.sadcas.org (accessed October 2, 2019).

SADCAS. n.d.-b. *What is SADCAS.* https://www.sadcas.org/what-sadcas (accessed October 2, 2019).

Serra, C. 2016. *The big data challenge for developing countries.* https://twas.org/article/big-data-challenge-developing-countries (accessed August 20, 2019).

Sharfstein, J. M. 2018. *The public health crisis survival guide: Leadership and management in trying times.* New York: Oxford University Press.

Silver, L., A. Smith, C. Johnson, J. Jiang, M. Anderson, and L. Rainie. 2019. Mobile connectivity in emerging economies. *Pew Research Center*, March 7, 2019.

Silverman, R. 2018. *Projected health financing transitions: Timeline and magnitude.* Washington, DC: Center for Global Development.

Sinha, K. 2011. Soon, bar code & unique no. On pill strips to check fakes. *The Times of India*, February 20, 2011. https://timesofindia.indiatimes.com/india/Soon-bar-code-unique-no-on-pill-strips-to-check-fakes/articleshow/7529728.cms (accessed February 13, 2020).

Smoke, P. 2015. *Accountability and service delivery in decentralizing environments: Understanding context and strategically advancing reform.* Paris, France: OECD.

Stevens, E. L., R. Timme, E. W. Brown, M. W. Allard, E. Strain, K. Bunning, and S. Musser. 2017. The public health impact of a publicly available, environmental database of microbial genomes. *Frontiers in Microbiology* 8:808.

Synalaf. 2013. *What is label rouge poultry?* http://www.volaillelabelrouge.com/en/what-is-label-rouge-poultry (accessed November 13, 2019).

The Global Health Network. 2019. Better research for better health. *Research Capacity Network.* https://rede.tghn.org/articles/better-research-better-health-university-oxford-and-fiocruz-partner-improve-health-research-and-capacity-development-globally (accessed December 8, 2019).

UNEP (United Nations Environment Programme) and FAO (Food and Agriculture Organization of the United Nations). 2014. *Voluntary standards for sustainable food systems: Challenges and opportunities.* Paper read at A Workshop of the FAO/UNEP Programme on Sustainable Food Systems, June 11–12, 2013, Rome, Italy.

UNIDO (United Nations Industrial Development Organization). 2016. *Strategic partnership between UNIDO and global food safety initiative announced.* https://www.unido.org/news/strategic-partnership-between-unido-and-global-food-safety-initiative-announced (accessed October 7, 2019).

USDA (U.S. Department of Agriculture). 2010a. *Food safety and inspection service strategic plan FY 2011–2016.* Washington, DC: USDA.

USDA. 2010b. *FSIS strategic data analysis plan for domestic inspection*. Washington, DC: USDA.

USDA. 2016. *Food safety and inspection service strategic plan 2017–2021*. Washington, DC: USDA.

USDA and Office of Inspector General. 2007. *Issues impacting the development of risk-based inspection at meat and poultry processing establishments*. Washington, DC: USDA.

Verhoeven, P., F. Sinn, and T. T. Herden. 2018. Examples from blockchain implementations in logistics and supply chain management: Exploring the mindful use of a new technology. *Logistics* 2(3):20.

Vought, R. 2019. *Memorandum for the heads of executive departments and agencies: Federal data strategy—a framework for consistency (m-19-18)*. https://www.whitehouse.gov/wp-content/uploads/2019/06/M-19-18.pdf (accessed August 28, 2019).

Wafula, F. N., E. M. Miriti, and C. A. Goodman. 2012. Examining characteristics, knowledge and regulatory practices of specialized drug shops in sub-Saharan Africa: A systematic review of the literature. *BMC Health Services Research* 12(1):223.

Wagner, A. K., J. D. Quick, and D. Ross-Degnan. 2014. Quality use of medicines within universal health coverage: Challenges and opportunities. *BMC Health Services Research* 14:357.

Waithira, N., B. Mutinda, and P. Y. Cheah. 2019. Data management and sharing policy: The first step towards promoting data sharing. *BMC Medicine* 17(1):80.

WBG (The World Bank Group). 2010. *Better regulation for growth: Governance frameworks and tools for effective regulatory reform*. http://documents.worldbank.org/curated/en/955811468330978599/Better-regulation-for-growth-governance-frameworks-and-tools-for-effective-regulatory-reform-institutions-for-regulatory-governance (accessed August 20, 2019).

WHO (World Health Organization). 2006. *A guide to healthy food markets*. Geneva, Switzerland: WHO. https://www.who.int/foodsafety/publications/healthy-food-market/en (accessed December 8, 2019).

WHO. 2014. *Regulatory system strengthening for medical products*. http://apps.who.int/medicinedocs/documents/s21456en/s21456en.pdf (accessed April 29, 2019).

WHO. 2016a. Annex 8: Collaborative procedure between the World Health Organization (WHO) prequalification team and national regulatory authorities in the assessment and accelerated national registration of WHO-prequalified pharmaceutical products and vaccines. In *WHO expert committee on specifications for pharmaceutical preparations*. Vol. 50. Geneva, Switzerland: WHO.

WHO. 2016b. Annex 11: Collaborative procedure in the assessment and accelerated national registration of pharmaceutical products and vaccines approved by stringent regulatory authorities. In *WHO expert committee on specifications for pharmaceutical preparations*. Vol. 50. Geneva, Switzerland: WHO.

WHO. 2017a. *WHO global surveillance and monitoring system for substandard and falsified medical products*. Geneva, Switzerland: WHO.

WHO. 2017b. *WHO Reference Group on Global Health Statistics (RGHS): Report & recommendations*. https://www.who.int/healthinfo/RGHS_MeetingReport_March2017.pdf?ua=1 (accessed August 20, 2019).

WHO. 2018. *Good practices of national regulatory authorities in implementing the collaborative registration procedures for medical products: Draft for comments*. https://www.who.int/medicines/areas/quality_safety/quality_assurance/02_08_2018_qas18_774_good_practices_of_NRAs_implementing_CRP_clean.pdf?ua=1 (accessed February 13, 2020).

WHO. 2019. *Report of an independent external review: Impact assessment of WHO prequalification and systems supporting activities*. https://www.who.int/medicines/Impact_assessment_WHO-PQ-RegSystems.pdf (accessed October 4, 2019).

WHO. n.d. *WHO Global Benchmarking Tool (GBT) for evaluation of national regulatory systems*. https://www.who.int/medicines/regulation/benchmarking_tool/en (accessed July 12, 2019).

Wyber, R., S. Vaillancourt, W. Perry, P. Mannava, T. Folaranmi, and L. A. Celi. 2015. Big data in global health: Improving health in low- and middle-income countries. *Bulletin of the World Health Organization* 93(3):203–208.

Yamagiwa, T. J. 2015. *El Salvador: The new law on medicines and its implementation.* Geneva, Switzerland: WHO.

Zanin, L. M., D. T. da Cunha, V. V. de Rosso, V. D. Capriles, and E. Stedefeldt. 2017. Knowledge, attitudes and practices of food handlers in food safety: An integrative review. *Food Research International* 100(Pt 1):53–62.

Zhang, Q., S. Liu, R. Liu, H. Xue, and Y. Wang. 2014. Food policy approaches to obesity prevention: An international perspective. *Current Obesity Reports* 3(2):171–182.

Appendix A

Committee Member Biographies

Catherine Woteki, PhD, RD (*Chair*), is a professor in the Department of Food Science and Human Nutrition at Iowa State University and a visiting distinguished institute professor at the University of Virginia's Biocomplexity Institute. From 2010 to 2016, she served as the chief scientist and the under secretary for the U.S. Department of Agriculture's (USDA's) Research, Education, and Economics mission area. In that role, she developed the Office of the Chief Scientist, established the USDA Science Council, and instituted the department's first scientific integrity and open data policies. She was called to lead scientific delegations to China and the first Meeting of Agricultural Chief Scientists held under the auspices of the G20. Dr. Woteki is an advocate for building the platforms needed to enhance domestic and international food and agricultural research. Prior to joining USDA, Dr. Woteki served as the global director of Scientific and Regulatory Affairs for Mars, Incorporated, where she managed the company's scientific policy on matters of health, nutrition, and food safety. From 2002 to 2005, she was the dean of agriculture and a professor of human nutrition at Iowa State University, and also the head of the Agricultural Experiment Station. Dr. Woteki served as the first under secretary for food safety at USDA from 1997 to 2001, where she oversaw the safety of meat, poultry, and egg products.

Lystra Antoine, JD, MBA, joined the Global Food Safety Partnership (GFSP) as its chief executive officer in August 2016. Under her leadership, the GFSP focused on (1) building capacity for science-based food control systems for all food exported and domestically consumed in developing countries; (2) convening key stakeholders to increase their involvement with and attention to food safety capacity building globally; and (3) increasing awareness for the importance of food safety for achieving the Sustainable Development Goals. For 4 years prior to joining the GFSP, Ms. Antoine worked as the global director for DuPont Pioneer's sustainable agriculture development efforts and was responsible for designing and leading the implementation of agriculture development initiatives that helped smallholder farmers improve their livelihoods and increase their contribution to the value chain. Ms. Antione spent 16 years at the World Bank prior to joining DuPont. She champions results-driven strategies to improve the human condition through safe, reliable, and sustainable food systems. Ms. Antione holds an MBA from SUNY Buffalo and a JD from the Georgetown University Law Center.

Mikel Arriola, JD, MPP, LLM, has a degree in law from the Universidad Anáhuac del Norte, a master in public policy and public administration from the London School of Economics and Political Science in London, England, as well as a master of laws from the University of Chicago. His career has been developed mainly in the public sector. In 2002, he was Banrural's litigation coordinator. From 2003 to 2005 he worked at Financiera Rural, where he held the positions of regulatory compliance manager and corporate deputy director of the General Directorate. In 2007, he joined the Ministry of Finance and Public Credit, an institution in which he was adviser to the secretary, the general director of Income Planning of the undersecretary of revenue and, as of 2009, the head of the Tax Legislation Unit of the undersecretary of revenue. In March 2011, he was appointed as federal commissioner for Protection against Health Risks of the Ministry of Health. In December 2012, he was confirmed to head Cofepris. In February 2016, Mr. Arriola was appointed the general director of the Mexican Institute of Social Security. Mr. Arriola is known for tightening prohibitions against so-called miracle weight loss treatments and for guidelines on the prevention of chronic disease.

Maria Elena Bottazzi, PhD, is the associate dean of the National School of Tropical Medicine; the co-section head and a professor of pediatric tropical medicine; a professor of molecular virology and microbiology at Baylor College of Medicine in Houston, Texas; and a distinguished professor in the Department of Biology at Baylor University in Waco, Texas. Dr. Bottazzi is also the co-director for the Texas Children's Hospital Center for Vaccine Development, a Product Development Partnership at Baylor College of Medicine. Dr. Bottazzi is an internationally recognized scientist with more than two decades of experience in translational research and vaccine development for emerging and neglected tropical diseases. In addition, her major interest is in the role of vaccines as control tools integrated into international public health programs and initiatives. As a global leader, she has received national and international awards, has authored more than 120 scientific papers, and has participated in more than 200 conferences worldwide. Currently, she is an Emerging Leader in Health and Medicine Scholar of the National Academy of Medicine, is the editor-in-chief of *Current Tropical Medicine Reports* (Springer, U.S.), and is the associate editor for *Public Library of Science (PLOS) Neglected Tropical Disease Journal*. Dr. Bottazzi's philosophy focuses on motivating and empowering peers and young generations of scientists building strong inter- and intra-relationships and positively contributing to scientific and global health effectiveness. Dr. Bottazzi has a bachelor's degree in microbiology and clinical chemistry from the National Autonomous University in Honduras, and a doctorate in molecular immunology and experimental pathology from the University of Florida. Her post-doctoral training in cellular biology was completed at the University of Miami and the University of Pennsylvania. Her academic tenure initiated at The George Washington University where she served for 11 years as an associate professor and a vice chair for administration in the Department of Microbiology, Immunology and Tropical Medicine prior to relocating to Houston in 2011.

Julie Caswell, MS, PhD, is a distinguished professor emeritus in the Department of Resource Economics at the University of Massachusetts (UMass) Amherst. Her research focuses on understanding the operation of domestic and international food systems, with particular interest in the economics of food quality and labeling, especially for safety and nutrition, and international trade. Dr. Caswell is a fellow of the Agricultural and Applied Economics Association (AAEA) and she is a past president of AAEA. She held a Fulbright Distinguished Lectureship at the University of Tuscia in Viterbo, Italy, in 2009. Dr. Caswell has served on several National Academies committees in the United States, including chairing the committee that published *Supplemental Nutrition Assistance Program: Examining the Evidence to Define Benefit Adequacy* in 2013, and she is currently serving on the Food and Nutrition Board. Dr. Caswell was senior associate dean for Education and Student Development in the College of Social and Behavioral Sciences at UMass Amherst. Dr. Caswell received her PhD jointly in agricultural economics and economics from the University of Wisconsin–Madison.

Clare Narrod, PhD, MS, is the director of the Risk Analysis Program at the Joint Institute for Food Safety and Applied Nutrition (JIFSAN) and leads the monitoring and impact effort associated with the evaluation of

JIFSAN's capacity building efforts. She received a PhD in energy management and environmental policy in 1997 and a master's degree in international development and appropriate technology from the University of Pennsylvania. From 1998 to 2000 she served as an American Association for the Advancement of Science Risk Analysis fellow at the U.S. Department of Agriculture (USDA). Prior to coming to JIFSAN, she worked at the International Food Policy Research Institute, USDA, and at the Food and Agriculture Organization of the United Nations. She has consulted for the World Bank and the Inter-American Institute for Cooperation on Agriculture. She has field experience in Brazil, China, Costa Rica, Ethiopia, Ghana, Hong Kong, India, Indonesia, Kenya, Mali, Mexico, Nigeria, Thailand, Vietnam, and Zambia. She has taught in China, Colombia, India, Malaysia, Russia, and the United States. She started her career in government, where she conducted and reviewed risk assessments and cost-benefit analyses of proposed and final rules for agency clearance associated with reducing the risk of animal and plant diseases and improving food safety. In addition to her work at JIFSAN, she is also a scientific advisory board member of the Institute for Food and Agricultural Literacy at the University of California, Davis, World Food Center and is on the board of directors for the Center for Foodborne Illness, Research & Prevention. In the past she has been a working group member on a Global Food Ethics Project at the Johns Hopkins Berman Institute for Bioethics, a member of the expert panel for a Global Regulatory Competency and Curricula, and a consensus committee member on the Institute of Medicine's study on Strengthening Core Elements of Regulatory Systems in Developing Countries.

Jonathan Quick, MD, MPH, is an adjunct professor of global health at the Duke Global Health Institute, Duke University. He is a senior fellow emeritus at Management Sciences for Health (MSH), where he previously served as president and chief executive officer from 2004 to 2017. In January 2017, he transitioned to the role of senior fellow. A family physician and health management specialist, Dr. Quick focuses on global health security. He is the author of *The End of Epidemics: The Looming Threat to Humanity and How to Stop It*. Dr. Quick was the director of essential drugs and medicines policy at the World Health Organization from 1996 to 2003. Prior to that, he served with MSH as the founding director of the drug management program/center for pharmaceutical management, then as a long-term advisor for the Afghanistan Health Sector Support Project and the Kenya Health Care Financing Project. He has worked in international health since 1978 and has carried out assignments in more than 70 countries in Africa, Asia, Latin America, and the Middle East. He is the senior editor of *Managing Drug Supply*, co-author of the *Financial Times Guide to Executive Health*, and has written over 100 other books, articles, and chapters. He is on the faculty of the Harvard Medical School Department of Global Health and Social Medicine and the Boston University School of Public Health, and is a fellow of the Royal Society of Medicine. He has a first degree from Harvard University, an MD with distinction in research, and an MPH from the University of Rochester.

Joshua Sharfstein, MD, is the vice dean for public health practice and community engagement and a professor of the practice in health policy and management at the Johns Hopkins Bloomberg School of Public Health. He is also the director of the Bloomberg American Health Initiative. Previously, Dr. Sharfstein served as the secretary of the Maryland Department of Health and Mental Hygiene, as the principal deputy commissioner of the U.S. Food and Drug Administration, and as the health commissioner of Baltimore City. He is an elected member of the National Academy of Medicine and the National Academy of Public Administration.

Markus Taussig, DBA, is an associate professor in the Management and Global Business Department at Rutgers Business School. Previous to his doctoral studies in strategy at Harvard Business School, Dr. Taussig lived in Vietnam for 11 years, where he researched development of that country's nascent private sector for the World Bank, The Asia Foundation, and various bilateral aid organizations. His academic work on business strategy in developing countries has been published in *American Political Science Review*, *Strategic Management Journal*, *Journal of Law, Economics and Organization*, *Journal of International Business Studies*, *Journal of East Asian Studies*, and *Business Horizons*. His more recent work on strategies for increasing regulatory compliance in developing countries is published in the *Academy of Management Journal* and in the *American Political Science Review* and was funded by the Jameel Poverty Action Lab, the World Bank, and the National University of Singapore. The work has received best paper awards from the Academy of Management's Public and Non-Profit Division and the International Association for Chinese Management Research. He is currently working on follow-up studies on regulatory compliance in Malaysia and Myanmar.

Raymond Wigenge, MSc, MBA, is a food technologist with more than 25 years of experience in food safety and regulation. He attained his MSc in food science and technology at Ghent University, Belgium, in 1997. He is also a holder of a BSc in food science and technology obtained at Sokoine University of Agriculture, Tanzania, in 1989. Other academic qualifications include an MBA obtained in 2013 at the Eastern and Southern African Management Institute, Arusha, Tanzania, and a diploma in animal production in 1980 in Mbeya, Tanzania. Since 1982, he has been employed as a public servant and served in different capacities, such as livestock extension officer, and agricultural tutor for 3.5 years. He has served in different roles, including food control officer, chief food inspector, zone offices and local government authority coordinator, and director of Food Safety for the Tanzanian Food and Drug Authority (FDA). During his career, he developed food regulations and guidelines, conducted food inspections, and was engaged in developing and implementing the food safety control system in Tanzania. He led development of the draft national food safety policy. He also designed a system for surveillance and investigation of foodborne diseases and acted as a key liaison between the Tanzania FDA and United Nations agencies such as the Food and Agriculture Organization, the World Health Organization, and the Codex Alimentarius Commission.

Veronika Wirtz, MSc, PhD, is an associate professor in the Department of Global Health at the Boston University School of Public Health, where she is also the director of the World Health Organization Collaborating Center in Pharmaceutical Policy. Her research focuses on health system strengthening and policy and program evaluations of medicines access and utilization. She is a visiting professor of the National Institute of Public Health (INSP) in Mexico and the coordinator of a student exchange program between the institutions of her affiliation. Her interest and expertise include medicines price analysis, generic medicines policies, quality use of medicines, access to medicines for noncommunicable diseases, and the role of the private sector to promote equitable access and efficient use of medicines in low- and middle-income countries. Between 2014 and 2016 she was the co-chair of The Lancet Commission on Essential Medicine Policies. From 2004 to 2012 she was a researcher and a lecturer at the National INSP in Mexico and a founding member and the head of the Medicines in Public Health Research Group, which is a multidisciplinary team of 15 experts in health economics, epidemiology, and social science carrying out pharmaceutical policy analysis in Mexico and Latin America. Over the last few years she has regularly taught short courses in pharmacoepidemiology and medicines utilization research at INSP in Mexico. She has worked as a technical adviser for various international organizations, among them the World Health Organization; the Pan American Health Organization; World Bank; the Global Fund to Fight AIDS, Tuberculosis and Malaria; the Bill & Melinda Gates Foundation; the Alliance for Health Systems and Policy Research; Health Action International; and the Ford Foundation. She has also worked with the Ministry of Health in Mexico on various program evaluations and capacity building initiatives. She is published widely in international peer-review journals such as *The Lancet*, *British Medical Journal*, *World Health Organization Bulletin*, *Health Policy and Planning*, *Health Policy*, *Value in Health*, *Social Science and Medicine*, and *Tropical*

Medicine and International Health. Since fall 2016 she has been the associate editor of *Health Systems & Reform*, a leading journal publishing health system and policy research. She received her training as a pharmacist from Albert-Ludwigs-University in Freiburg, Germany, and her master in clinical pharmacy and a PhD from the University of London.

Prashant Yadav, MBA, PhD, is a globally recognized scholar in the area of health care supply chains. He is a visiting fellow at the Center for Global Development, an affiliate professor of technology and operations management at INSEAD, and a lecturer at the Harvard Medical School. He is the author of many peer-reviewed scientific publications, and his work has also been featured in prominent print and broadcast media, including *The Economist*, *The Financial Times*, *Nature*, and the BBC. Outside academia, Dr. Yadav works closely with governments and global organizations in the area of policy and investment strategy design for health care supply chains. Until recently Dr. Yadav was the strategy leader–supply chain at the Bill & Melinda Gates Foundation. Dr. Yadav serves on the advisory boards of many global organizations and social enterprises. He has been invited for expert testimony on the issue of medicine supply chains in the U.S. Congress and legislative bodies in other countries. He was a commissioner on the Lancet Commission on Essential Medicines and has been a member of multiple National Academy of Medicine Expert Committees. He was the chair of the Market Dynamics Advisory Group of the Global Fund to Fight AIDS, Tuberculosis and Malaria, Geneva, and the co-chair of procurement and supply chain management at the Roll Back Malaria Partnership. Dr. Yadav's research papers have been the recipient of the best paper awards from the Production and Operations Management Society, INFORMS, and other professional societies. He was inducted as a Chartered Fellow of the Chartered Institute of Logistics and Transport in 2011. Before his current role, Dr. Yadav was vice president of health care at the William Davidson Institute at the University of Michigan and a faculty member at the Ross School of Business at the University of Michigan. Before that, he was a professor of supply chain management at the Massachusetts Institute of Technology (MIT)-Zaragoza International Logistics Program and a research affiliate at the MIT Center for Transportation and Logistics.

Appendix B

Public Meeting Agendas

COMMITTEE ON STRONGER FOOD AND DRUG REGULATORY SYSTEMS ABROAD

The Keck Center, 500 Fifth Street, NW
Washington, DC 20001

JANUARY 8, 2019
ROOM 100

8:30	Breakfast available

SESSION 1—CLOSED
BIAS AND CONFLICT OF INTEREST
OVERVIEW OF STUDY

9:00–12:00	Bias and Conflict of Interest Discussion Overview of National Academies' Processes Review Study Statement of Task and Timeline
12:00–1:00	Lunch
1:00–1:30	Overview of Report Communications
1:30–1:45	Break

SESSION 2—OPEN
CAPACITY AND INSTITUTIONAL DEVELOPMENT

1:45–2:15	The Global Benchmarking Tool **Mike Ward,** *Coordinator*, Regulatory Systems Strengthening, Essential Medicines and Health Technologies, World Health Organization
2:15–2:45	Institutional Development and Financing **Analia Porrás,** *Unit Chief*, Medicines and Health Technologies, Health Systems and Services, Pan American Health Organization
2:45–4:30	Panel Discussion on Management of the Regulatory Agency **Mikel Arriola,** *Committee Member*, Moderator **Lembit Rago,** *Secretary General*, Council for International Organizations of Medical Sciences **Kenneth Hartigan-Go,** *Associate Professor, Department of Strategic Management & Head* **Stephen Zuellig,** Graduate School of Development Management, Asian Institute of Management **Dali Yang,** *William C. Reavis Professor of Political Science & Senior Advisor to the President and the Provost on Global Initiatives*, University of Chicago
4:30	Adjourn
6:00	Working dinner for committee and staff at Rasika restaurant

JANUARY 9, 2019
ROOM 100

8:30	Breakfast available in Room 105

SESSION 3—OPEN
CAPACITY CONTINUED, TECHNICAL ASSISTANCE AND LOCAL MARKETS

9:00	Welcome **Catherine Woteki**, *Committee Chair*
9:05–9:30	Benchmarking for Food Safety **Steven Jaffee**, *Lead Rural Development Specialist*, World Bank (by phone)
9:30–10:00	Technical Assistance and Accountability **Renata Clarke**, *Senior Food Safety and Quality Officer*, Food Safety and Quality Unit, Food and Agriculture Organization (FAO) (by video)
10:00–10:15	Break
10:15–11:45	Panel Discussion on Donor and Private-Sector Engagement **Jono Quick**, *Committee Member*, Moderator **Kelley Cormier**, *Division Chief*, Bureau for Food Security, *U.S. Agency for International Development*[1] **Nuri Gras**, *Executive Secretary*, Chilean Food Safety and Quality Authority **Dilip Shah**, *Secretary General*, Indian Pharmaceutical Alliance (by video) **Jude Nwokike**, *Director, Promoting the Quality of Medicines*, U.S. Pharmacopeia
11:45–12:45	Lunch for committee, speakers, and staff in Room 105
12:45–2:15	Panel Discussion on Product Quality and Local Markets **Joshua Sharfstein**, *Committee Member*, Moderator

[1] Dr. Cormier was unable to attend due to the federal government shutdown.

Delia Grace, *Veterinary Epidemiologist*, International Livestock Research Institute
Spencer Henson, *Professor*, University of Guelph
Elizabeth Pisani, *Associate Professor*, School of Health Policy and Management, Erasmus University
Gugu Mahlangu, *Director General*, Medicines Control Authority of Zimbabwe

2:15–2:30 Break

SESSION 5—OPEN
HARMONIZATION AND REGIONAL COOPERATION

2:30–4:00 Panel Discussion on Regional Cooperation
Prashant Yadav, *Committee Member*, Moderator
Lisa Indar, *Program Manager*, *Tourism and Health*, Caribbean Public Health Agency
Jarbas Barbosa, *Assistant Director*, Pan American Health Organization
Larry Liberti, *Executive Director*, Centre for Innovation in Regulatory Science
Gugu Mahlangu, *Director General*, Medicines Control Authority of Zimbabwe
Anban Pillay, *Deputy Director General for Health Regulation and Compliance*, National Department of Health (by phone)

SESSION 6—CLOSED
COMMITTEE DELIBERATIONS

4:00–5:00 Committee Deliberations

5:00 Adjourn

Committee on Stronger Food and Drug Regulatory Systems Abroad

Academy of Sciences of Costa Rica
Los Yoses, San Pedro, Costa Rica

FEBRUARY 25, 2019

9:00–9:15	Welcome and Introductions **Catherine Woteki,** *Committee Chair*
9:15–9:30	Opening Remarks **Pedro Leon,** Academy of Sciences of Costa Rica
9:30–9:45	Introduction to Food and Drug Administration Latin America **Katherine Serrano,** *Director, Latin America Office,* Food and Drug Administration
9:45–10:00	Break

SESSION 1—OPEN
FOOD SAFETY SYSTEMS

10:00–10:25	Food and Agriculture Organization and World Health Organization Food Control Assessment Tool **Marisa Caipo,** *Food Safety and Quality Officer,* FAO Regional Office for Latin America and the Caribbean
10:25–10:50	New Food Safety Management System for Ecuador **Rommel Anibal Betancourt Herrera,** *General Coordinator of Food Safety,* Agency for Regulation and Control of Plant and Animal Health (AGROCALIDAD)
10:50–11:15	The Effects of the U.S. Food Safety Modernization Act on Local Markets **Ana Marisa Cordero,** *Specialist,* Agricultural Health and Food Safety, Inter-American Institute for Cooperation on Agriculture

11:15–11:40 The Effect of Codex Standards on Local Food Markets
Tatiana Cruz Ramirez, *Head, Department of Technical Regulation and Codex*, Ministry of Economy, Industry and Commerce, Costa Rica

11:40–12:40 Lunch

12:40–2:20 Panel Discussion on Food Safety (All Session 1 Speakers)
Mikel Arriola, *Moderator*

- *Latin American countries generally have large agricultural sectors that employ a lot of people. Do you see a tension between food regulation for the promotion of trade and food regulation for domestic consumption?*
- *Most food safety systems emphasize choosing priorities based on risk. What are the barriers to doing this?*
- *What factors aid or hold back your ability to work with other countries in the region on foodborne disease, outbreaks, and emergencies? How would you say this has changed over the last 5 to 10 years?*

2:20–2:35 Break

SESSION 3—OPEN
MEDICAL PRODUCT SAFETY SYSTEMS

2:35–3:05 Strengthening Medicines Regulation in Central America
Jose Vicente Coto Ugarte, *Regional Consultant, Medicines*, Pan American Health Organization

3:05–3:35 Approval and Registration of Biotherapeutics
Emilio Medina, *Technical and Scientific Director*, Development and Research Processes, National Polytechnical Institute of Mexico
Mayra Perez-Tapia, *Executive Director & Research Professor*, Unit for Development and Research in Bioprocesses, National Polytechnical Institute of Mexico

3:35–4:05 Licensing and Inspection of Drug Manufacturer, Import, and Wholesale
Jean Carlo Apuy, *Enforcement*, College of Pharmacy of Costa Rica (COLFAR)

4:15 Adjourn

FEBRUARY 26, 2019

9:00–9:15 Welcome
Catherine Woteki, *Committee Chair*

SESSION 4—OPEN
INDUSTRY AND CONSUMER PERSPECTIVES

9:15–11:00 Panel Discussion on Openness and Industry's Role in Regulatory Systems
Maria Elena Bottazzi, *Moderator*

- *How would you describe the relationship between public confidence in your products and the strength of the regulatory agency?*
- *How do you see industry's role in building strong regulatory agencies in the countries where you work?*
- *Can you share examples of times when you found regulatory action to be predictable and objective and times when it was not?*
- *What is your experience of the regulatory agencies' ability to respond to new technologies?*

Rivelino Flores, *Director of Regulatory Affairs and Innovation*, National Chamber of the Pharmaceutical Industry
Monique Collaço de Moraes Stávale, *Vice Director of Quality*, Bio-Manguinhos, Oswaldo Cruz Foundation
Paula Vargas, *Regulatory Leader*, Pfizer, Central America and the Caribbean
Lissy Cruz, *Regulatory Manager*, Fedefarma
Mario Montero, *Executive Vice President*, Cámara Costarricense de la Industria Alimentaria, the food industry association of Costa Rica

11:00–11:15 Break

11:15–11:45 Open Sharing of Government Data
Ana Gabriel Zuniga, Hivos Latin America

11:45–12:15 Information, Education, and Communication with Consumers
Carolina Paz, Center for Consumer Defense, El Salvador

12:15–1:15 Lunch

SESSION 5—OPEN
THE CHALLENGES FACING REGULATORY AGENCIES

In their brief introductory comments, speakers are asked to describe their agency, its responsibilities, when it was founded, and how it is funded.

1:15–1:40 Staff and Agency Development Planning[2]
Maria Angelica Sanchez Herrera, *former Head, Office of International Affairs*, National Institute for Drug and Food Surveillance (Invima)

1:40–1:55 Introduction to ARSA
Iris Galeano, *Commissioner*, Sanitary Regulatory Agency (ARSA) Honduras

1:55–2:10 Introduction to ARCSA
Juan Carlos Galarza, *Executive Director*, National Agency for Health Regulation, Control, and Surveillance (ARCSA), Ecuador

2:10–2:25 Introduction to Anvisa
Dirceu Barbano, *former Director General*, National Health Surveillance Agency (Anvisa) Brazil

2:25–2:35 Break

[2] Rescheduled from previous day.

2:35-4:05 Panel Discussion with Session 6 Speakers
Joshua Sharfstein, *Moderator*

- *What are the main challenges facing your agency with regard to food safety, medicine, and vaccine safety?*
- *Would you say staff retention is a problem, and if so, what do you think would help retain talented workers?*
- *Is the food and drug regulatory agency a priority for heads of government, ministers of health, and ministers of finance? If not, what might persuade them to make it one?*
- *What are the main barriers to persuading heads of government to invest in regulatory systems?*

4:05 Adjourn Public Meeting

SESSION 6—CLOSED COMMITTEE DEBRIEF

4:05–5:00 Committee Debrief

Committee on Stronger Food and Drug Regulatory Systems Abroad

National Academy of Sciences,
2101 Constitution Avenue, NW, Washington, DC 20418

APRIL 3, 2019
ROOM 125

SESSION 1—OPEN
BUILDING SYSTEMS ON RISK

9:00–9:15	Welcome and Introductions **Catherine Woteki**, *Committee Chair*
9:15–9:45	Reforms at FSSAI **Pawan Agarwal**, *Chief Executive*, Food Safety and Standards Authority of India (by video)
9:45–10:15	Risk Based Food Safety in Ethiopia **Barbara Kowalcyk**, *Assistant Professor, Food Science and Technology*, The Ohio State University
10:15–10:30	Break

SESSION 2—OPEN
RAISING THE PROMINENCE OF REGULATORY SYSTEMS

10:30–10:50	Regulatory Systems and Public Health **Carlos Santos Burgoa**, *Professor*, *Department of Global Health*, The George Washington University
10:50–11:10	The Hidden Costs of Neglecting Medicines Regulation **Mac Lumpkin**, *Deputy Director Integrated Development*, Bill & Melinda Gates Foundation (by video)
11:10–11:30	Industry Action to Improve Regulatory Systems **Uy Hong Nguyen**, *Regulatory and External Affairs Director*, Abbott Nutrition, Vietnam
11:30–12:30	Lunch in cafeteria

12:30–12:50 Driving Investment in the Regulatory Agency
Javier Guzman, *Technical Director*, *Pharmaceuticals and Health Technologies*, Management Sciences for Health

12:50–2:15 Panel Discussion: All Morning Speakers
Catherine Woteki, *Moderator*

- *What messages would best encourage investment in regulatory systems? How would the messages differ for donors, ministers of health, and ministers of finance?*
- *Can you describe the communication strategy that regulatory agencies could use to improve understanding of their work by the public and a strategy to better advocate for support from their ministers?*

2:15–2:30 Break

SESSION 3—OPEN
DONOR MOTIVATORS AND THE FUTURE OF AID

2:30–2:50 Gavi Transition Financing
Santiago Cornejo, *Senior Specialist*, *Immunization Financing*, Gavi

2:50–3:10 Facilitating Safer Food Systems
Kelley Cormier, *Division Chief*, *Inclusive Market Development*, U.S. Agency for International Development

3:10–3:30 U.S. Agency for International Development Support for Drug Regulatory Systems: Reasons for Involvement and Changes Over Time
Lisa Ludeman, *Senior Pharmaceutical Management Technical Advisor*, U.S. Agency for International Development

3:30–3:50 Managing Risk and Benefits in Medicines Systems: The Example of Dolutegravir
Alain Prat, *Team Lead, Quality Assurance*, The Global Fund

3:50–5:00 Panel Discussion: Session 3 Speakers
Julie Caswell, Moderator

- *Would you agree that food and drug regulatory systems have not been a donor priority in the past? Could you explain why that might be or what might change it?*
- *How do you expect the substance and manner of donor involvement in health to change over the next 10 years?*

5:00 Adjourn

Appendix C

Call for Comments

The National Academies Committee on Stronger Food and Drug Regulatory Systems Abroad seeks comment on how emerging technologies can help food or drug regulatory agencies, especially those in low- and middle-income countries, better protect product safety. Of interest are examples of technologies that

1. support quality in informal markets;
2. reduce the cost of regulatory work; or
3. improve efficiency.

The committee also seeks comment on the challenges of using these technologies. Anyone wishing to submit a comment should email the committee at fooddrugregsys@nas.edu. We request that comments be submitted before **June 14, 2019**. All comments will be filed for public access.

Appendix D

Ensuring Safe Foods and Medical Products Through Stronger Regulatory Systems Abroad

BOX D-1
Statement of Task from the 2012 Report

The U.S. Food and Drug Administration (FDA) has requested that the Institute of Medicine convene a consensus study to assist the FDA in:

(A) Identifying the core elements of needed pharmaceutical, biologics, medical device, and food safety regulatory systems development in developing countries; and in
(B) Prioritizing these needs and recommending a strategic approach to the FDA's moving forward to address regulatory capacity needs in the context of globalization.

In addition to identifying and prioritizing the core elements of regulatory systems development, the consensus study would also identify:

(C) Potential areas in which progress could be made in a 3- to 5-year time frame;
(D) Priorities for FDA engagement;
(E) Areas to which others (bilateral donors, development banks, foundations, academia, industry, and non-governmental organizations) are best suited to contribute; and
(F) How the FDA might best "partner" with these other institutions to bring to their efforts the expertise that the FDA has in an effort to leave a more sustainable "footprint" from both their and the FDA resource commitments.

Specific questions to be explored by the Consensus Study Committee shall at least include:

1. What critical issues do developing country regulatory authorities face, and how are they prioritized?

2. In what ways do they participate in standard-setting processes, organizations, and harmonization efforts?
3. What issues do they face in utilizing/implementing standards in a sustainable way?
4. What are the core elements of their regulatory systems, and are there others that should be considered?
5. What are the major gaps in systems, institutional structures, workforce, and competencies?
6. In what ways could those gaps be addressed?
7. In what ways could the U.S. FDA help address those gaps?
8. In what ways could others (as delineated above) help meet those gaps?
9. In what ways could the FDA partner with others to help meet those gaps?
10. What recommendations have already been put forward to strengthen regulatory systems?
11. What obstacles exist to implement those recommendations?
12. What steps could be taken to remove those obstacles?
13. What incentives and controls would be needed to support efforts?

Given that "developing countries" include a heterogeneous group of about 150 low- and middle-income countries, for the purposes of this study emphasis will be given to understanding in some depth the issues for a limited number of countries that currently are or are expected to soon become major pharmaceutical and agricultural trading partners with the United States (e.g., Mexico, Brazil, South Africa, India, Thailand, and China).

SOURCE: IOM, 2012.

TABLE D-1
Recommendations from the 2012 Report

Type	Recommendation
International Action	**Recommendation 5-1:** In the next 3 to 5 years, international and intergovernmental organizations should invest more in strengthening the capacity of regulatory systems in developing countries. The United States should work with interested countries to add it to the G20 agenda. Investments in international food and medical product safety should be a significant and explicitly tracked priority at development banks, regional economic communities, and public health institutions. International organizations should provide assistance to achieve meaningful participation of developing country representatives at international harmonization and standardization meetings.
	Recommendation 5-2: In emerging economies, national regulatory authorities, regulated industry, and industry associations should engage in open and regular dialogue to exchange scientific and technical information before policies are written and after they are implemented. Starting in the next 3 to 5 years, these regulatory authorities should identify third parties, such as science academies, to convene the three pillars of a regulatory system—government, industry, and academia—in ongoing discussion to advance regulatory science, policy, and training.
	Recommendation 5-3: Countries with stringent regulatory agencies should, within the next 18 months, convene a technical working group on sharing inspection reports with the longer-term goal of establishing a system for mutual recognition of inspection reports.
	Recommendation 5-4: Industry associations should, over the next 3 years, define an acceptable protocol for sharing of internal inspection results among their members. After agreeing on the methods, they should regularly share their results among their members.
	Recommendation 5-5: Starting in the next 5 years USAID, FDA, CDC, and USDA should provide (both directly and through WHO and FAO) technical support for strengthening surveillance systems in developing countries. This technical support could include development and sharing of surveillance tools, protocols for foodborne disease surveillance and post market surveillance of medical products, and training of national regulatory authority staff and national experts.
Domestic Action	**Recommendation 6-1:** The FDA should use enterprise risk management to inform its inspection, training, regulatory cooperation, and surveillance efforts. Enterprise risk management should apply to the agency's entire operation, and it should incorporate a number of set criteria, such as country of manufacture or production, volume and type of product, facility inspection history, and trends or data shared from other regulatory authorities.

Type	Recommendation
	Recommendation 6-2: The FDA should develop an information and informatics strategy that will allow it to do risk-based analysis, monitor performance metrics, and move toward paperless systems. In the next 3 to 5 years, the FDA should propose, in all its international harmonization activities, a standardized vocabulary, a minimum data set to be collected, and the frequency of data collection.
	Recommendation 6-3: The FDA should facilitate training for regulators in developing countries. The purpose is workforce training and professional development through an ongoing, standing regulatory science and policy curriculum. In the next 3 to 5 years, the FDA should broaden the scope of FDA University to educate FDA staffers on international compliance with its regulations. In the long term, the FDA should consider the options the committee puts forth in this chapter.
	Recommendation 6-4: U.S. policy makers should integrate food and medical product safety objectives into their international economic development, trade, harmonization, and public health work. To this end, the FDA should lead in the development and adoption of international and harmonized standards for food and medical products.
	Recommendation 6-5: The FDA, which currently requires one-up, one-back track-and-trace requirements for food, should, in the next year, hold a multi-sector, international, public workshop on applying them to medicines, biologics, and (when appropriate) to devices.
	Recommendation 6-6: Starting in the next 2 years, the FDA and USDA should implement Cooperative Research and Development Agreements and other programs to encourage businesses and academia to research and develop innovations for low-cost, appropriate fraud prevention, intervention, tracking, and verification technologies along the supply chain.
	Recommendation 6-7: The FDA should ensure an adequate mix of incentives to importers of food and medical products that are confirmed to meet U.S. regulatory standards. One such promising initiative is the 2-year FDA Secure Supply Chain pilot program. The FDA should evaluate this program immediately after its pilot phase (scheduled to end in 2014). The program should be expanded, if successful, to include a greater number of importers and food.
	Recommendation 6-8: Over the next 10 years, U.S. government agencies should work to strengthen the ability of those harmed by unsafe food and medical products to hold foreign producers and importers liable in civil lawsuits.

SOURCE: IOM, 2012.

TABLE D-2
Gaps in Regulatory Systems in Developing Countries

	Gaps	
Problems	Food Systems	Medical Product Systems
Adherence to international standards	• Lack of awareness of public health risks • Lack of funding and expertise • Lack of adherence to manufacturing and agricultural standards	• Problems adhering to quality standards • Lack of funding for quality-control laboratories • Challenges implementing good manufacturing practices • Inconsistent adherence to international research standards
Controlling supply chains	• Lack of good transportation and storage • Inadequate equipment	• Inefficient post-market surveillance • Lack of optimal storage • Lack of modern information technology and supply chain management
Infrastructure	• Lack of laboratories, manufacturing, and market infrastructure • Lack of information technology and communication • Lack of reliable electricity, water sanitation, and pest control • Lack of adequate roads	
Laws	• Outdated or poorly coordinated laws governing food or drug safety • Lack of enforcement of existing regulations	
Workforce	• Too few regulatory staff • Insufficient technical training for staff • Problems retaining staff	

TABLE D-2 Continued

	Gaps
Institutional fragmentation	• No clear assignment of responsibilities or established protocol for enforcement, unclear chain of command • Lack of established communication channels between and within agencies
Surveillance	• Passive foodborne disease surveillance • Lack of food chain security and information sharing • Lack of pharmacovigilance systems • Passive or spontaneous adverse event reporting • Lack of active and post-market surveillance
Communication	• Lack of communication within a regulatory authority and across government agencies that share regulatory responsibility • Lack of communication between regulatory authorities and regulated industry • Lack of communication between the regulatory authority and the public • Lack of communication with counterpart regulatory agencies abroad
Political will	• Competing priorities and limited budgets • Corruption and lack of accountability

SOURCE: IOM, 2012.

BOX D-2
Essential Elements of Food and Medical Product Regulatory Systems

Government is the foundation for a strong regulatory system. As the national standard-setting body, governments:

- use science and risk as a basis for developing policy;
- participate in international cooperation and harmonization of standards;
- make ethical decisions; and
- recognize, collect, and transmit evidence when breaches of law occur.

A food and medical product regulatory system integrates:

- product safety through good manufacturing, clinical, laboratory, and agricultural practices;
- staff development and training for employees;
- monitoring and evaluation of product quality using laboratories;
- inspection and surveillance of products throughout the supply chain;
- risk assessment, analysis, and management; and
- emergency response.

Protecting the public's health is crucial in a food and medical product regulatory system. The system needs to quickly communicate information to the public in emergencies to ensure the public's safety.

SOURCE: IOM, 2012.

REFERENCE

IOM (Institute of Medicine). 2012. Ensuring safe foods and medical products through stronger regulatory systems abroad. Washington, DC: The National Academies Press.